FOGSI FOCUS
Endometriosis: Current Trends

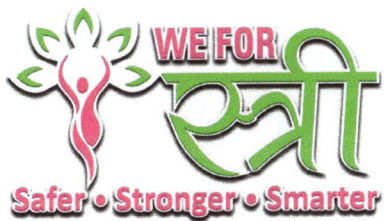

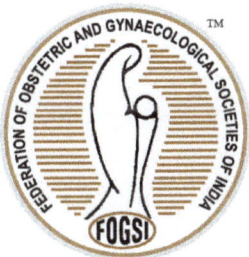

Federation of Obstetric and Gynaecological Societies of India (FOGSI)

FOGSI FOCUS
Endometriosis: Current Trends

Editor-in-Chief

Nandita Palshetkar MD FCPS FICOG FRCOG (UK)
President of FOGSI 2019
Scientific Director, Bloom IVF
Professor of Obstetrics and Gynecology
Dr DY Patil Medical College, Hospital and Research Centre
Navi Mumbai, Maharashtra, India

Editor

Kuldeep Jain MD Fellow ART (Singapore)
IVF Consultant and Gynae Laparoscopic Surgeon
Director, KJIVF and Laparoscopy Centre, Delhi
Chairperson, Endometriosis Committee

Co-Editors

Sudha Prasad MBBS MS FICOG FICMCH
IVF Coordinator at IVF and Reproductive Biology Centre
Department of Obstetrics and Gynecology
Lok Nayak Hospital and Maulana Azad Medical College
Delhi, India

T Ramani Devi MD DGO FICS FICOG
Consultant, Obstetrician & Gynaecologist and Reproductive Medicine
Vice President Elect, South Zone FOGSI 2020
Department of Obstetrics and Gynaecology
Ramakrishna Medical Centre LLP
Trichy, Tamil Nadu, India

Fessy Louis T DGO DNB FAGE MNAMS DPS MICOG FICOG
Senior Consultant and Associate Professor
Department of Reproductive Medicine and Surgery
Amrita Fertility Centre, AIMS
Amrita Institute of Medical Sciences
Kochi, Kerala, India

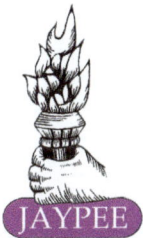

JAYPEE BROTHERS MEDICAL PUBLISHERS
The Health Sciences Publisher
New Delhi | London

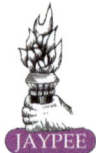 **Jaypee Brothers Medical Publishers (P) Ltd**

Headquarters
Jaypee Brothers Medical Publishers (P) Ltd
4838/24, Ansari Road, Daryaganj
New Delhi 110 002, India
Phone: +91-11-43574357
Fax: +91-11-43574314
Email: jaypee@jaypeebrothers.com

Overseas Office
J.P. Medical Ltd
83, Victoria Street, London
SW1H 0HW (UK)
Phone: +44 20 3170 8910
Fax: +44 (0)20 3008 6180
E-mail: info@jpmedpub.com

Website: www.jaypeebrothers.com
Website: www.jaypeedigital.com

© 2020, Jaypee Brothers Medical Publishers

The views and opinions expressed in this book are solely those of the original contributor(s)/author(s) and do not necessarily represent those of editor(s) of the book.

All rights reserved. No part of this publication may be reproduced, stored or transmitted in any form or by any means, electronic, mechanical, photocopying, recording or otherwise, without the prior permission in writing of the publishers.

All brand names and product names used in this book are trade names, service marks, trademarks or registered trademarks of their respective owners. The publisher is not associated with any product or vendor mentioned in this book.

Medical knowledge and practice change constantly. This book is designed to provide accurate, authoritative information about the subject matter in question. However, readers are advised to check the most current information available on procedures included and check information from the manufacturer of each product to be administered, to verify the recommended dose, formula, method and duration of administration, adverse effects and contraindications. It is the responsibility of the practitioner to take all appropriate safety precautions. Neither the publisher nor the author(s)/editor(s) assume any liability for any injury and/ or damage to persons or property arising from or related to use of material in this book.

This book is sold on the understanding that the publisher is not engaged in providing professional medical services. If such advice or services are required, the services of a competent medical professional should be sought.

Every effort has been made where necessary to contact holders of copyright to obtain permission to reproduce copyright material. If any have been inadvertently overlooked, the publisher will be pleased to make the necessary arrangements at the first opportunity. The **CD/DVD-ROM** (if any) provided in the sealed envelope with this book is complimentary and free of cost. **Not meant for sale.**

Inquiries for bulk sales may be solicited at: jaypee@jaypeebrothers.com

FOGSI FOCUS Endometriosis: Current Trends

First Edition: **2020**
ISBN: 978-93-89188-84-4

Office Bearers of Team FOGSI 2019

President	Dr Nandita Palshetkar
Secretary General	Dr Jaydeep Tank
Vice President (West Zone)	Dr Rajendrasingh Pardeshi
Vice President (West Zone)	Dr Haresh Doshi
Vice President (North Zone)	Dr Sudha Prasad
Vice President (East Zone)	Dr Rajat Mohanty
Vice President (South Zone)	Dr Aswath Kumar
Deputy Secretary General	Dr Madhuri Patel
Treasurer	Dr Suvarna Khadilkar
Joint Treasurer	Dr Parikshit Tank
Joint Secretary	Dr Ameya Purandare
Immediate Past President	Dr Jaideep Malhotra
President Elect	Dr Alpesh Gandhi

Chairpersons of the Committees

Adolescent Health	Dr Girish Mane
Clinical Research	Dr Meena Samant
Endocrinology	Dr Pratik Tambe
Endometriosis	Dr Kuldeep Jain
Endoscopic Surgery	Dr B Ramesh
Ethics and Medicolegal	Dr Geetendra Sharma
Family Welfare	Dr Shobha Gudi
Food Drugs Medico Surgical Equipment	Dr Vidya Thobbi
Genetics and Fetal Medicine	Dr Mandakini Pradhan
HIV/AIDS	Dr Mrutyunjay Mohapatra
Imaging Science	Dr Meenu Agarwal
Infertility	Dr Asha Baxi
International Academic Exchange	Dr Varsha Baste
MTP	Dr Bharti Maheshwari
Medical Education	Dr Abha Singh
Medical Disorders in Pregnancy	Dr Komal Chavan
Midlife Management	Dr Rajendra Nagarkatti
Oncology	Dr Bhagyalaxmi Nayak
Perinatology	Dr Vaishali Chavan
Practical Obstetrics	Dr Sanjay Das
Public Awareness	Dr Kalyan Barmade
Quiz	Dr Sebanti Goswami
Safe Motherhood	Dr N Palaniappan
Breast	Dr Sneha Bhuyar
Sexual Medicine	Dr Sudha Tandon
Urogynaecology	Dr Nita Thakre
Young Talent Promotion	Dr Vinita Singh

Contributors

Abha Majumdar MS
Director and Head
Centre of IVF and Human Reproduction
Institute of Obstetrics and Gynaecology
Sir Ganga Ram Hospital
New Delhi, India

Asha R Rao MD
Chief Consultant
Department of Infertility
RAO Hospital
Coimbatore, Tamil Nadu, India

Bharti Jain DNB Fellowship in ART
Senior Radiologist and ART Consultant
Department of Reproductive Medicine
KJIVF and Laparoscopy Centre
Delhi, India

Damodar R Rao MS
Associate Director and Senior Consultant
Department of Endogynaecology
RAO Hospital
Coimbatore, Tamil Nadu, India

Dhivya Sethuraman MD
Associate Professor
Department of Obstetrics and Gynaecology
SRM Medical College
Trichy, Tamil Nadu, India

Fessy Louis T MBBS DGO Dip NB FICOG
Senior Consultant & Associate Professor
Department of Reproductive Medicine
Amrita Institute of Medical Science
Kochi, Kerala, India

Kuldeep Jain MD Fellow ART (Singapore)
IVF Consultant and Gynae Laparoscopic Surgeon
Director, KJIVF and Laparoscopy Centre, Delhi
Chairperson, Endometriosis Committee
Delhi, India

Maansi Jain MS Fellowship in Reproductive
Medicine and Surgery (Singapore)
Consultant, ART
Department of Reproductive Medicine
KJIVF and Laparoscopy Center
Delhi, India

Meenakshi Dua MD
Senior Consultant
Southend Fertility and IVF
New Delhi, India

M Preethi MS
Resident Fellowship in Endogynaecology
Department of Endogynaecology
RAO Hospital
Coimbatore, Tamil Nadu, India

Nandita Palshetkar MD FCPS FICOG
Medical Director
Bloom IVF
Mumbai, Maharashtra, India
President, FOGSI (2019)
President, IAGE (2017-18)
Chairperson, MSR (2017-18)
Vice President, AMOGS (2016-18)

Neeti Tiwari MD FICOG
Consultant
Centre of IVF and Human Reproduction
Institute of Obstetrics and Gynaecology
Sir Ganga Ram Hospital
New Delhi, India

Nutan Jain MS
Director
Department of Obstetrics & Gynae
Vardhman Trauma & Laparoscopy Centre Pvt Ltd
Muzaffarnagar, UP, India

Parul Kotdawala MD Dip Pelviscopy FICOG FICMCH
Consultant
Zydus Hospital
Endoscopy Surgeon
Department of Obstetrics and Gynecology
VS Hospital & NHL Municipal Medical College
Ahmedabad, Gujarat, India

Parvathy T MS Mch
Assistant Professor
Department of Reproductive Medicine
Amrita Institute of Medical Science
Kochi, Kerala, India

Pratik Tambe MD FICOG
ART Consultant and Gynaec Endoscopic Surgeon
Chairperson, FOGSI Endocrinology Committee (2017-19)
Managing Council Member, MOGS
Managing Council Member, MSR, AMC, IAGE (2015-18)
Mentor, MOGS Youth Council
Mumbai, Maharashtra, India

Riddhi Desai MS PGDMLS Dip in Endoscopy (Pune)
Dip in Office Hysteroscopy (Italy)
Consultant
Advanced Multispecialty Hospital
Mumbai, Maharashtra, India

Rohan Palshetkar MS
Consultant Fertility Specialist
Bloom IVF
Mumbai, Maharashtra, India

Santwan B Mehta MS FMAS FRM
Endoscopic Surgeon
Zydus Hospital
Ahmedabad, Gujarat, India

Saumya Prasad MS
Senior Resident
Department of Obstetrics and Gynecology
Maulana Azad Medical College
New Delhi, India

Sonia Malik DGO MD FICOG FIAMS
Director and HOD
Southend Fertility & IVF
New Delhi, India

Sudha Prasad MS FICOG FICMCH
IVF Coordinator at IVF and Reproductive Biology Centre
Department of Obstetrics and Gynecology
Lok Nayak Hospital and Maulana Azad Medical College
New Delhi, India

Surveen Ghumman MD
Director and Head
Department of IVF & Reproductive Medicine
Max Multispeciality Hospitals
New Delhi, India

T Ramani Devi MD DGO FICS FICOG
Consultant
Obstetrician and Gynaecologist and
Reproductive Medicine
Vice President Elect, South Zone FOGSI 2020
Department of Obstetrics and Gynaecology
Ramakrishna Medical Centre LLP
Trichy, Tamil Nadu, India

President's Message

My Dear FOGSI Members
Greetings from FOGSI !

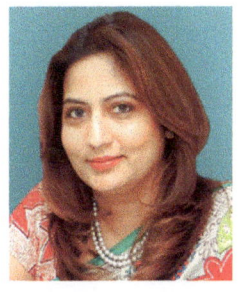

Endometriosis affects an estimated 10 to 15% of the female population. It has various presentations and degrees of severity. In its most severe form this disease is very debilitating for patients, compromising not just their fertility but also their social, professional, and personal life. It has become a major public health problem associated with high monetary costs and a significant decline in productivity. Endometriosis is not acknowledged in society, and hence is underdiagnosed and so is undertreated.

This FOGSI Focus on endometriosis is a welcome addition to all the literature available on endometriosis. It provides a balanced blend of all aspects of endometriosis like history and a discourse on pathogenesis, along with descriptions of clinical symptomatology, medical and surgical therapeutic approaches, and offers suggestions for holistic care of patients.

The editor of this FOGSI Focus Dr Kuldeep Jain and Co-editors, Dr Sudha prasad, Dr Ramani Devi and Dr Fessy Luice T have compiled a publication on endometriosis which is holistic and will provide us with a practical and evidence-based approach which will be of great value to clinicians and trainees.

Nandita Palshetkar
President, FOGSI

Preface

"He who knows Endometriosis, knows Gynecology"
—**Sir William Osler**

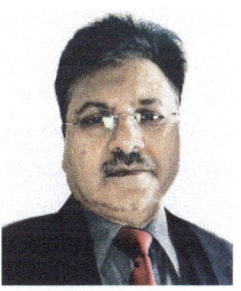

Endometriosis is a common and debilitating condition that can have a significant impact on the quality of life of the sufferer. It is a disease of controversy/complexity, chronic/multi-factorial, progressive/recurrent, not malignant but behaves like one and difficult to diagnose and treat. Once diagnosed clinically and by various imaging modalities, there is a wide variation of interventions available for treatment ranging from ovarian suppression with hormonal agents to radical excisional surgery. This suggests that the condition is heterogeneous and that there is a lack of consensus over optimal management. Laparoscopy remains gold standard and is the best tool for diagnosis, treatment and follow-up evaluation of endometriosis. Endometriosis affects over 176 million women worldwide and 6–10% of women of reproductive age are affected. An incidence of 2.37–2.49/1000 has also been reported with a relative prevalence of 6–8% in the general population. There is a higher incidence of infertile women. 25% of patients undergoing ART are affected and 20–40% of these patients show ovarian endometriosis.

It is estimated that 25–35% of infertile women have endometriosis while 30–50% of women with endometriosis have infertility. Eight per cent of women in ART programs have the primary diagnosis of endometriosis made. In a review of 61 women with endometriosis 48 of which underwent controlled ovarian hyperstimulation showed the need for higher total dose or ampoules of gonadotropins to produce an average of 3 metaphase II eggs, 50% fertilization rate but pregnancy rates were lower in those with moderate to severe disease. Fecundability is 0.20 in unaffected women but 0.02–0.20 in women with endometriosis. Another report indicates a fecundity of 0.15–0.20 per month in normal couples but 0.02–0.10 in untreated women with endometriosis and infertility. Therefore in women with stage III-IV monthly probability to conceive is 2–10% vs. 15–25% in healthy couples.

Choice of management depends on the presenting symptoms, age, fertility history and progression and recurrence. If the primary symptom is pain and fertility is not the issue, definitive surgery with as much cytoreduction is possible is the treatment of choice, however if the fertility is the issue or patient is young, a conservative approach is recommended. Medical treatments that inhibit ovulation have been found to be effective in reducing pain in 80–90% of women. Medical therapy, however, is not cytoreductive and pain recurrence is frequent after treatment withdrawal. Moreover, side effects and costs discourage long-term use and it does not improve pregnancy rates in women with associated infertility.

For generations it has been taught that abdominal hysterectomy and removal of both ovaries is the definitive surgery for endometriosis. However, our understanding of the disease has evolved. Technological advances in camera optics and electrosurgical devices and improved surgical experience, combined with the limitations of medical treatment, now make operative laparoscopy the preferred management choice for a considerable proportion of women.

In vitro fertility (IVF) is the appropriate treatment especially in the presence of tubal function compromise, male factor or failure of other treatments. IVF is an effective treatment in women with infertility and endometriosis. IVF is appropriate treatment especially if there are multiple causes of infertility and/or other treatments have failed. Surgery may have some role in mild endometriosis and cases with large endometriomas as surgical treatment may improve outcomes. IVF is a useful and effective procedure to treat infertile women with endometriosis although its success rate could be impaired by the disease itself. If there is a negative effect, the oocyte quality more than the endometrium seems to be affected, this may explain why outcomes are better in women with endometriosis who have recipient cycles. Some large data bases did not show adverse effect on pregnancy rates (SART and HFEA) in women with endometriosis.

Considering the complex nature of endometriosis, dilemmas debates and controversies involved in the diagnosis, management and follow-up, and newer suggested molecules for medical management as well as changing concepts for improving the fecundity and cumulative pregnancy rates in ART. This edition of FOGSI FOCUS is planned to cover all areas from diagnosis, etiopathology to advances in medical management to managing deep infiltrative endometriosis to different newer stimulation protocols and fertility preservation and decision making in infertile couples, and I am happy that all contributors have put in their best effort to compile various chapters in such a way that they are clinically useful and easy to understand.

I am thankful to FOGSI president Dr Nandita Palshetkar for giving me the opportunity to bring this FOGSI FOCUS in my last working year as chairperson, endometriosis committee. I am also thankful to my Co-editors Dr Sudha Prasad, Dr Ramani Devi and Dr Fessy Louise T for giving there valuable inputs to complete this work in time. I acknowledge the timely submission of very high quality academic material by all contributing authors.

I express my deep appreciation to Dr Prateek Tambe for extending all possible help to bring out this work in time. I will be only too happy if the chapters in this volume of FOGSI focus are of benefit to all practicing gynecologist of country in helping to treat all endometriosis patients coming to them for help.

Kuldeep Jain

Contents

1. **Newer Insights in Etiopathogenesis of Endometriosis** 1
   Saumya Prasad, Sudha Prasad

2. **Endometriosis in Adolescent: Clinical Challenges** 6
   M Preethi, Damodar R Rao, Asha R Rao

3. **Imaging in Endometriosis** 13
   Bharti Jain, Maansi Jain

4. **Medical Management of Endometriosis and Adenomyosis—What's New** 17
   Sonia Malik, Meenakshi Dua

5. **Adenomyosis and Assisted Reproductive Technology** 24
   Kuldeep Jain, Maansi Jain, Bharti Jain

6. **Müllerian Anomalies and Endometriosis** 29
   T Ramani Devi, Dhivya Sethuraman

7. **Stimulation in Endometriosis and Adenomyosis: Is It Different?** 37
   Abha Majumdar, Neeti Tiwari

8. **Tips of Surgery in Endometriosis** 42
   Nutan Jain

9. **Rectosigmoid Endometriosis/Deep Infiltrative Endometriosis** 48
   Parul Kotdawala, Santwan B Mehta

10. **Fertility Prevention and Endometriosis: What is the Status?** 58
    Surveen Ghumman

11. **Scar Endometriosis—Preservation Strategies and Management** 62
    Pratik Tambe, Riddhi Desai

12. **Endometriosis and Infertility** 66
    Rohan Palshetkar, Nandita Palshetkar

13. **Surgery before In Vitro Fertilization: What is the Evidence and Recommendations?** 73
    Fessy Louis T, Parvathy T

Index 79

CHAPTER 1

Newer Insights in Etiopathogenesis of Endometriosis

Saumya Prasad, Sudha Prasad

INTRODUCTION

Endometriosis is a chronic, estrogen-dependent inflammatory, heritable disorder which is characterized by growth of endometrial tissue in sites other than the uterine cavity, most commonly in the pelvic cavity, including the ovaries, the uterosacral ligaments, and the pouch of Douglas.[1] The disease affects approximately 10% of the women in reproductive age group.[2] Despite not being at their normal anatomical positions these heterotopic endometrial tissues remain responsive to the circulating estrogen levels. Just like their normal anatomical counterparts these grow and shed with each cycle of ovulation. The shed endometrial glands and stroma incite strong chronic inflammatory response via cytokines leading to production of prostaglandins and ultimately fibrosis.[3]

Clinical diagnosis of endometriosis is often difficult due to the wide spectrum of symptoms which are mostly nonspecific. There are no pathognomonic features necessary and sufficient to define endometriosis. Endometriosis is typically defined by its histology: extra uterine lesions consisting of endometrial glands, stroma, and hemosiderin-laden macrophages.[4] Based on location and depth, lesions are further described as superficial, ovarian endometrioma or deep endometriosis. Visual observation through transvaginal sonography (Fig. 1), laparoscopy (Fig. 2), and histopathological sampling are the gold standards.[5] The most common complaints in endometriosis patients are dysmenorrhea (79%) and chronic pelvic pain (69%).[6]

The pathogenesis of endometriosis is still not definitive, though many theories have been proposed including retrograde menstruation, coelomic metaplasia, embryonic cell rest, lymphovascular metastasis, and stem cell.

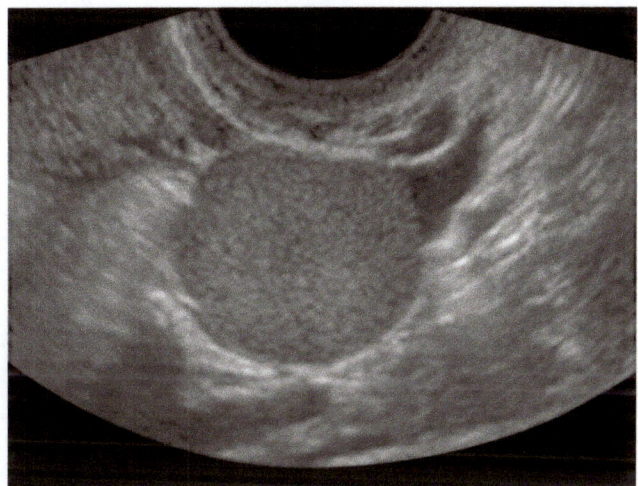

Fig. 1: Left-sided endometrioma on transvaginal sonography.

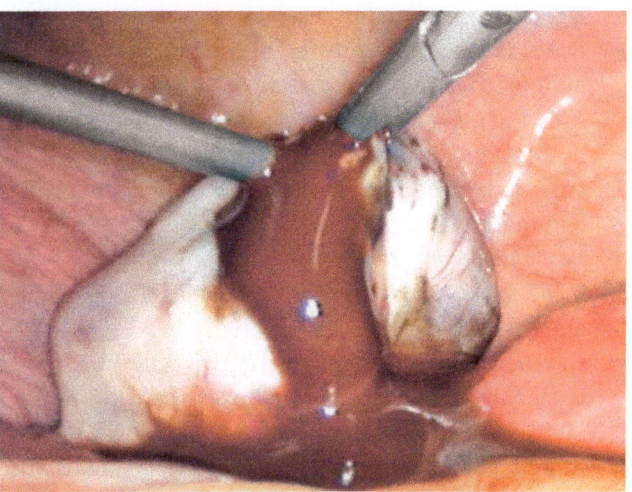

Fig. 2: Left-sided endometrioma on laparoscopy.

PATHOGENESIS OF ENDOMETRIOSIS

Theories of Endometriosis[7]

- *Sampson theory of retrograde menstruation*: This is the most popular theory. This theory explains retrograde flow of menstrual blood from uterus through fallopian tubes into the peritoneal cavity. Endometrial fragments get implanted onto peritoneal surface at dependent sites like ovaries, uterosacral ligaments and pouch of Douglas (Figs. 3 and 4). Although this theory can explain pelvic endometriosis, it fails to explain distant endometriosis. Moreover, implantation of endometrial tissue has been shown to be dependent more on genetic predisposition and hormonal environment and not merely on retrograde menstruation.

  This theory is supported by laparoscopic findings of menstrual blood components during perimenstrual period.
- *Halban's theory of lymphatic spread*: This theory can explain endometriosis inflicting pelvic lymph nodes. This theory proposes that endometrial tissue can metastasize through the draining lymph channels of uterus to the lymph nodes.
- *Meyer and Ivanoff theory of coelomic metaplasia*: Mesothelial cells from peritoneal and ovarian surfaces may undergo metaplasia to endometrial tissue. This can occur due to chronic irritation by the menstrual blood. Alternatively, Müllerian remnants in form of primordial cells might get trapped into the peritoneum of posterior pelvic wall during embryogenesis and later undergo metaplasia under high serum estrogen levels. Stem cells can also transform into endometrial tissue under hyperestrogenic state.
- *Direct implantation theory*: This theory postulates that endometrial cells can directly get implanted at new sites and grow. These sites can be abdominal scar after hysterotomy, cesarean section or myomectomy and episiotomy scars. However, this theory does not explain endometriosis at other sites.
- *Vascular theory*: This is the least explained theory but it can explain endometriosis at distant sites like lungs and brain (Fig. 5).
- *Genetic theory*: A multifactorial or polygenic inheritance is seen in patients of endometriosis. There is 6–7 times increased risk in first degree relatives. However, such inheritance is observed in merely 10% of patients. Also concordance for endometriosis is frequently observed in monozygotic twin-pairs. Predisposed women are more prone to grow endometrium at ectopic sites. Genes responsible for increased susceptibility have been found to be *EMX2*—a transcriptional factor encoding proteins for reproductive tract development and *PTEN*—a tumor suppressor gene responsible for malignant transformation to endometroid adenocarcinoma in ovarian endometriosis. Both these genes are located within or near *20p13* locus. Other genes implicated in pathogenesis of endometriosis are those encoding for interleukin (IL)-15, glycodelin, Dickkopf-1, semaphoring E, aromatase, progesterone receptor (PR), and multiple angiogenic factors.
- *Biomolecular theory*: Patients of endometriosis have an impaired immune system response, increased production of cytokines and proinflammatory mediators, increased overall angiogenic activity, excessive estrogen production, and progesterone resistance. Peritoneal

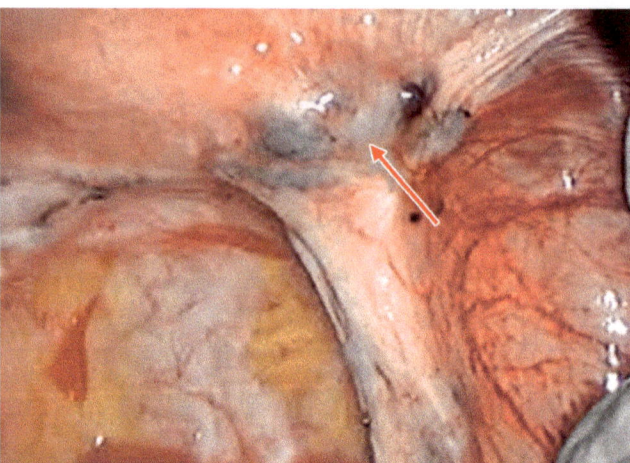

Fig. 3: Endometriosis involving uterosacral ligament (red arrow).

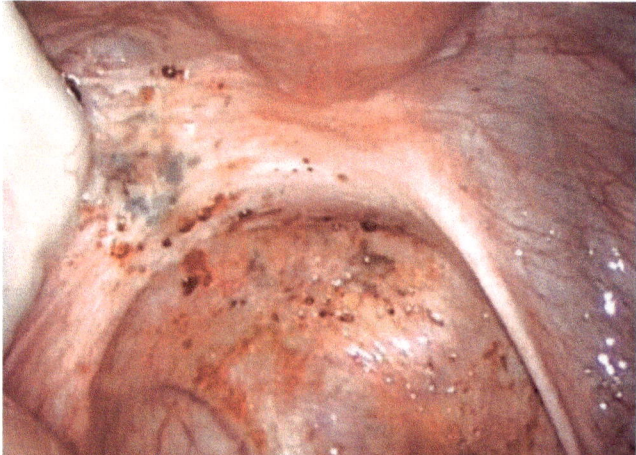

Fig. 4: Burnt out areas of mild endometriosis.

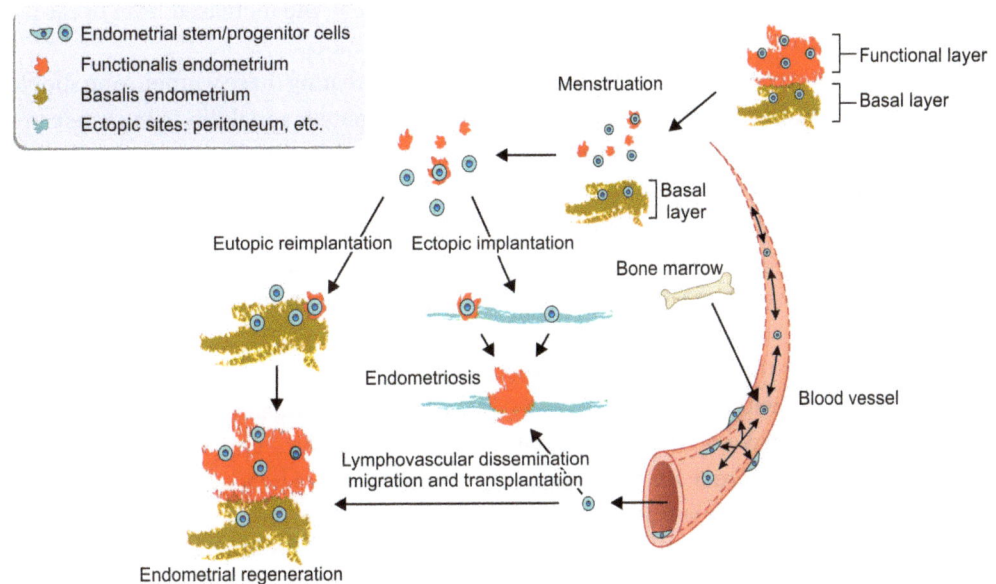

Fig. 5: Lymphovascular dissemination of endometriotic cells.

macrophages phagocytize menstrual debris in normal women. Ectopic endometriotic implants do not undergo phagocytosis and apoptosis due to decreased expression of metalloproteinase, *CD36*, and increased production of dissolved intercellular adhesion molecule-1. In patients of endometriosis due to subclinical peritoneal inflammatory response, activated macrophages secrete increasing amounts of proinflammatory cytokines like IL-1, IL-6, IL-8, monocyte chemoattractant protein (MCP)-1, regulated on activation, normal T-cell expressed and secreted (RANTES), tumor necrosis factor (TNF)-α, TNF-β, integrins, and angiogenic factors. These cytokines promote growth of endometrium at ectopic sites and makes them more resistant to apoptosis by further triggering release of more prostaglandins and proangiogenic vascular endothelial growth factor (VEGF). In addition, these cytokines have detrimental impact on sperm motility. They promote phagocytosis of sperms and can interfere with fertilization process. Prostaglandins also increase activity of *aromatase (p450arom)* and the production of tissue estrogen promoting an overall hyper estrogenic milieu.

The most important factor in the pathogenesis of endometriosis is estrogen dysregulation and progesterone resistance. In normal females, there is dominance of alpha subtypes of estrogen receptors (ER-α). In endometriosis beta subtypes of estrogen receptors (ER-β) overwhelm alpha receptors. It is postulated that epigenetic mutation by hypomethylation of the CpG cluster of estrogen receptor genes is responsible for this change from alpha to beta dominance. The increased levels of ER-β suppress production of ER-α. This in turn reduces the formation of PRs, resulting in progesterone resistance in endometriosis. ER-β also regulates cell cycle progression and leads to increased proliferation of endometriotic cells.

- *Environment theory*: The most important toxin are dioxins (e.g. *TCDD-2,3,7,8-tetracholorodibenzo-p-dioxin*). These are by-products of industrial processing and often enter our body through food chain. These promote somatic mutation of endometrium by acting as transcription factors promoting increased ILs synthesis, activation of *cytochrome P450,* and alteration of tissue remodeling.

Among these existing theories on endometriosis pathogenesis, Sampson's retrograde menstruation theory is scientifically proven, easy to understand and widely acceptable.[8] The theory is also supported by laparoscopic findings where menstrual blood components were found in peritoneal cavity. Consistently, Müllerian remnant theory also describes that spreading of primordial cells across the posterior pelvic wall may transform into endometrial tissue when exposed to high-level estrogenic stimulus.[9]

Technological progress in molecular biology has increased the interest in genetic polymorphism identification and its involvement in endometriosis development. A polygenic inheritance is seen in patients of endometriosis.[10] The endometriotic tissue is sensitive to estrogen and progesterone. The two estrogenic receptor isoforms (ER-α, ER-β) are codified by two different genes (*ESR*1 and *ESR*2) with different tissue-specific distributions; they can join to different ligands and activate different genes for transcription. The influence of ESR1 has been correlated with severe endometriosis in various studies.[11] There is 6–7 times increased risk in first degree relatives. Endometriotic genes responsible for increased susceptibility have been found to be *EMX2*—a transcriptional factor encoding proteins for reproductive tract development.[12]

Implantation failure in patients with endometriosis is directly associated with low endometrial *HOXA10* levels. *EMX2*, a mammalian ortholog of Drosophila empty spiracles gene, is a transcription factor which is necessary for Müllerian duct and renal development.[13] High endometrial *HOXA10* expression occurs in mid-late secretory phase of the menstrual cycle. Conversely, it is observed that high levels of *EMX2* mRNA were reported in the proliferative in association with the low levels of *HOXA10*.[13]

Long noncoding RNAs (lncRNAs) are a class of noncoding RNAs with at least 200 nucleotides.[14] The major pathway involved in up regulating mRNAs in eutopic vs. normal endometrium included cytokine–cytokine receptor interaction, hypoxia-inducible factor-1 signaling, mitogen-activated protein kinase (MAPK) signaling, apoptosis, NF-κB signaling, and focal adhesions. Enrichment of mRNAs in innate immune response indicated correlation between immune factors and endometriosis.[15]

Endometriosis patients have an impaired immune system response, increased production of cytokines and proinflammatory mediators, increased overall angiogenic activity, excessive estrogen production, and progesterone resistance. Endometriotic cells have the ability to avoid immune surveillance, granting them easier implantation and growth in ectopic places. Cytokines like TNF-α, TNF-β, and integrins promote growth of endometrium at ectopic sites and makes them resistant to apoptosis.[16] Whereas estrogen dysregulation and progesterone resistance are important factor in the pathogenesis of endometriosis. In healthy females, alpha subtype of estrogen receptors is dominant while beta subtype of estrogen receptor is seen in endometriosis. It is postulated that epigenetic mutation by hypomethylation of the CpG cluster of estrogen receptor genes is responsible for this change from alpha to beta dominance.[17] The increased level of ER-β suppresses production of ER-α.

While treating these women, one should always keep in mind that genetic variability in humans can cause numerous mutations which alter at cellular and molecular level and maintain the development of illness. Understanding the role of genetics, epithelial progenitor cells will allow a more targeted and effective therapeutic approach to this poorly understood disorder.

REFERENCES

1. Vercellini P, Viganò P, Somigliana E, et al. Endometriosis: pathogenesis and treatment. Nat Rev Endocrinol. 2014;10(5):261-75.
2. Acién P, Velasco I. Endometriosis: A disease that remains enigmatic. ISRN Obstet Gynecol. 2013;(4):242149.
3. Garai J, Molnar V, Varga T, et al. Endometriosis: harmful survival of an ectopic tissue. Front Biosci. 2006;11(1):595-619.
4. Tabbara SO, Covell JL, Abbitt PL. Diagnosis of endometriosis by fine-needle aspiration cytology. Diagn Cytopathol. 1991;7(6):606-10.
5. Woodward PJ, Sohaey R, Mezzetti TP Jr. Endometriosis: radiologic-pathologic correlation. Radiographics. 2001;21(1):193-216.
6. Fauconnier A, Chapron C, Dubuisson JB, et al. Relation between pain symptoms and the anatomic location of deep infiltrating endometriosis. Fertil Steril. 2002;78(4):719-26.
7. Vinatier D, Orazi G, Cosson M, et al. Theories of endometriosis. Eur J Obstet Gynecol Reprod Biol. 2001;96(1):21-34.
8. Holoch KJ, Lessey BA. Endometriosis and infertility. Clinic Obstet Gynecol. 2010;53(2):429-38.
9. Suardika A, Pemayun TG. New insights on the pathogenesis of endometriosis and novel non-surgical therapies. J Turk Ger Gynecol Assoc. 2018;19(3):158-64.
10. Simpson JL, Bischoff FZ, Kamat A, et al. Genetics of endometriosis. Obstet Gynecol Clin. 2003;30(1):21-40.
11. Giudice LC, Burney RO, Becker C, et al. Genetics and genomics of endometriosis. In: Leung, Peter CK, Jie Q (Eds). Human Reproductive and Prenatal Genetics. Cambridge, MA: Academic Press; 2019. pp. 399-426.
12. He B, Ni ZL, Kong SB, et al. Homeobox genes for embryo implantation: From mouse to human. Animal Models Exp Med. 2018;1(1):14-22.
13. Daftary GS, Troy PJ, Bagot CN, et al. Direct regulation of β3-integrin subunit gene expression by HOXA10 in endometrial cells. Mol Endocrinol. 2002;16(3):571-9.

14. Taft RJ, Pang KC, Mercer TR, et al. Non-coding RNAs: Regulators of disease. J Pathol. 2010;220(2):126-39.
15. Vigano P, Gaffuri B, Somigliana E, et al. Expression of intercellular adhesion molecule (ICAM)-1 mRNA and protein is enhanced in endometriosis versus endometrial stromal cells in culture. Mol Hum Reprod. 1998;4(12):1150-6.
16. Chegini N, Williams RS. Cytokines and growth factor networks in human endometrium from menstruation to embryo implantation. In: HA Joseph (Ed). Cytokines in Human Reproduction. New York: Wiley-Liss; 2000. pp. 93-132.
17. Koukoura O, Sifakis S, Spandidos DA. DNA methylation in endometriosis. Mol Med Rep. 2016;13(4):2939-48.

CHAPTER 2

Endometriosis in Adolescent: Clinical Challenges

M Preethi, Damodar R Rao, Asha R Rao

INTRODUCTION

Endometriosis was frequently described as an enigmatic condition due to many unanswered questions and controversies in its pathogenesis, diagnosis, and management. Endometriosis was once believed to occur in teenagers rarely and was thought to affect women in later reproductive years. With increasing awareness of both healthcare professionals and general population, it is now well revealed that endometriosis affects significant teenagers.

After introduction of keyhole surgery since 1980s, endometriosis is recognized as a disease that affects adolescent and young women, whereas in the beginning it was believed that it was rare in younger age group.

Endometriosis prevalence in adolescents undergoing keyhole surgery for chronic pelvic pain is reported to be between 19% and 73%. To our surprise rarely, endometriosis has also been notified in premenarchal girls with some breast development. Diagnosis of adolescent endometriosis is often delayed in the adolescent girls for more than 6–8 years if high index of suspicion is not there.

Several factors have been described for endometriosis, whereas no single theory can explain the cause of symptoms. Genetic factors may play a role, whereas lifestyle characteristics and environmental factors can also be related to the development of the disease.

The raising concern on this topic is because this diagnosis of condition is quite challenging.

- Presenting symptoms of adolescent endometriosis is persistent chronic pelvic pain, in spite of treatment with medical management like either hormonal contraceptives or pain killers.
- In almost 60–70% of adults with endometriosis, symptoms started even before the women reached 20s.
- In spite of using an oral contraceptive or pain killers, these girls tend to have more school absentees during their menses and also take leave more for a longer period of time to treat severe primary dysmenorrhea.
- Several symptoms, which are associated with gastrointestinal tract, are seen with these adolescent girls like constipation, diarrhea, nausea, and vomiting.
- Appearance of adolescent endometriosis may be different from adult endometriosis and also deeper lesions seem to be rare.
- There is no evidence whether the treatment for adolescent endometriosis may prevent disease progression in their later life.

RISK FACTORS

Most commonly obstructive type Müllerian anomalies are known to be associated with increased risk of endometriosis in teenagers. It may be due to increased retrograde menstruation. After surgical correction of obstruction, spontaneous resolution of such endometriosis has been reported. There is a familial association in adolescent endometriosis similar to adult endometriosis.[1,2]

SYMPTOMS

Major presenting symptoms of endometriosis in adolescence are chronic pelvic pain (27–96%) and dysmenorrhea (18–100%). Severe acyclic pain tends to be more common in these teens than in adults. Other symptoms are urinary symptoms, gastrointestinal symptoms, pelvic mass, irregular menses, dyspareunia, subfertility, migraine, and depression or anxiety. Adolescents should be offered a pain diary in order to document frequency and pain characters.[2,3]

HISTORY

Past medical history, family history, and physical examination are necessary for evaluation and management of adolescents with a possible endometriosis. Several other pathologies, such as appendicitis, pelvic inflammatory disease, bowel disease, Müllerian anomalies or outflow obstruction, musculoskeletal disorders, hernias and psychosocial complaints should be excluded prior to diagnose adolescent endometriosis.[3,4]

EXAMINATION

Inspection of the girl should be done for possible estrogen-dependent body configuration with peripheral fat distribution and also for breast and pubic hair development according to the Tanner system.

A patent outflow tract should be evaluated in these teen adolescents by placing a Q-tip into the vaginal canal. This is very helpful to exclude a possible transverse vaginal septum, vaginal agenesis or agenesis of the lower vagina. For virgo adolescents pelvic examination cannot be performed; hence, rectal-abdominal examination is done. Importance should be given for diagnosis of both diffuse and focal pelvic tenderness.[3,5]

Investigations

Imaging is very helpful in these girls. Ultrasonography and magnetic resonance imaging (MRI) will perform anatomical evaluation, but are not specific for diagnosing endometriosis.

Transvaginal Ultrasound

In case of suspected endometriosis, transvaginal ultrasound is necessary to investigate even if the pelvic and/or abdominal examination is normal so as to identify endometriomas and deep endometriosis involving the bowel, bladder or ureter. In virgins where transvaginal scan is not appropriate, consider for a transabdominal ultrasound imaging of the pelvis.[6]

Magnetic Resonance Imaging

According to some studies, *MRI* can detect endometrial implants with a sensitivity as high as 60% but due to its high cost, it is better not to use pelvic MRI as the primary investigation to diagnose endometriosis in women with symptoms and signs of endometriosis. It is better to consider pelvic MRI only to assess the extent of deep endometriosis involving the bowel, bladder or ureter.[6]

CA 125

Cancer antigen (CA 125) is very sensitive, but they are not specific, thus, is not so helpful in the diagnosis of adolescent endometriosis. If in case of coincidentally reported increased serum CA 125 level is available, then a raised serum CA 125 (that is, 35 IU/mL or more) may be consistent with endometriosis. Despite endometriosis may be present even with a normal serum CA 125 (less than 35 IU/mL).[1,6]

ROLE OF DIAGNOSTIC LAPAROSCOPY

Adolescents with severe symptoms should be appropriately evaluated by *diagnostic laparoscopy* where standard treatment for pelvic pain or dysmenorrhea is not effective. Endometriosis should be staged by using the revised criteria of the American Society of Reproductive Medicine-based classification system. Thus, during a diagnostic laparoscopy, it is always better to take a biopsy of suspected endometriosis, in order to confirm the diagnosis of endometriosis (but be aware that a negative histological result does not exclude endometriosis).[6,7]

Large numbers of lesions in adolescent populations with endometriosis are atypical red lesions and majority of these lesions were correlated with severe dysmenorrhea and abdominal pain, nausea, constipation and diarrhea due to increased production of prostaglandins (Figs. 1A and B).

Some study had reported peculiar atypical red vascular lesions in 60% of adolescents teens compared to only 20% of nonadolescents. Clear lesions are common in adolescent endometriosis but often it is difficult to visualize and evaluate these lesions. Peritoneal defects or windows are common manifestations of adolescent endometriosis (Fig. 2).[7,8]

NATURAL COURSE OF ENDOMETRIOSIS IN TEENAGERS

The natural course of endometriosis in adolescents has always been a matter of debate. In adults spontaneous resolution, particularly of superficial lesions, has been reported, but in teenagers, some authors reported progression of endometriosis lesions in few patients who underwent a second-look laparoscopy after ablative therapy of endometriosis. Due to this reason, some authors have a belief that teenage endometriosis is a progressive disease.[3,9]

MEDICAL TREATMENT

Nonsteroidal Anti-inflammatory Drugs

Due to high prevalence of severe dysmenorrhea in teenagers, it is always better to treat these young girls with

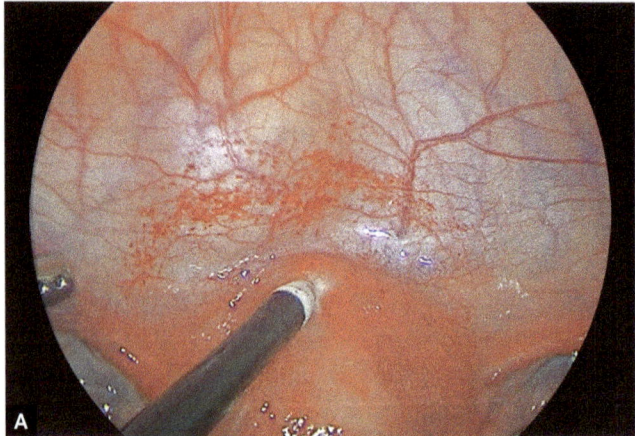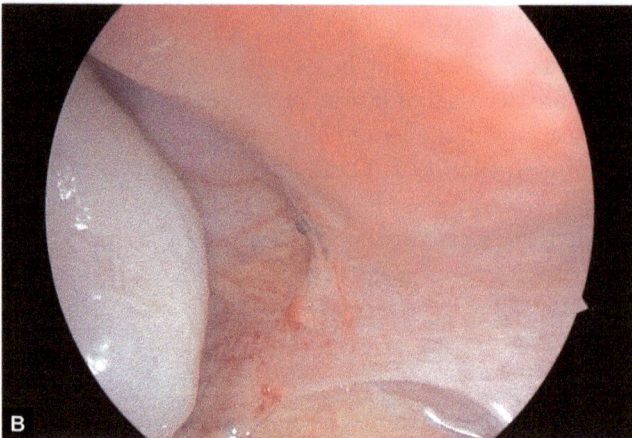

Figs. 1A and B: Peculiar atypical red vascular lesions.
Courtesy: Rao Hospital, Coimbatore.

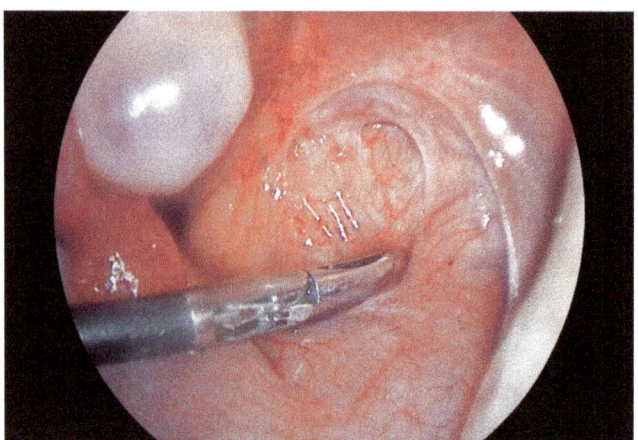

Fig. 2: Peritoneal windows in endometriosis.
Courtesy: Rao Hospital, Coimbatore.

the classical approach of nonsteroidal anti-inflammatory drugs (NSAIDs), oral contraceptive pills, and/or paracetamol.[2,5] Thus, it has to be remembered that both primary dysmenorrhea and endometriosis-associated pain will respond to these kinds of therapies whereas symptomatic improvement does not rule out endometriosis. Hence, it is always better to communicate this message to both the teenager and her parents/caregivers. In this sort of approach it is expected that the symptoms will improve and avoid a significant number of further unnecessary investigations including gonadotropin-releasing hormone agonist (GnRHa) or laparoscopy. But it is also better to explain to parents or caregivers that the symptoms of endometriosis may be masked due to NSAIDs, thus allowing the condition to progress further.

Hormonal Treatment

In those women with suspected or confirmed endometriosis, hormonal treatment may reduce pain, but it has no permanent negative effect on subsequent fertility. Thus, it is better to offer hormonal treatment [e.g., the combined oral contraceptive (COC) pill or a progestogen] to women with recurrent endometriosis. If the pain is not responding to the COC or NSAIDs treatment, then there is a high likelihood of endometriosis. Hence, before starting options of medical management like GnRH analogs or dienogest (DNG) diagnosis with diagnostic laparoscopy may be considered as an option.

Levonorgestrel Intrauterine System

In adolescents who are sexually active, levonorgestrel intrauterine system (LNG-IUS) may be effective alternative for those who have endometriosis-associated pain. Due to lack of evidence in its use among teenagers, it may not be considered as an acceptable option among teenagers. Thus, it may not be used as a first-line empirical treatment option.[1,4]

GnRHa

Those teenagers who have surgically confirmed disease, treatment with GnRHa may be considered as an option. However, overuse of GnRHa in teenagers who are at the critical stage of achieving the peak bone density is of concern. In spite of this, some studies suggest that GnRHa can be an alternate option for treatment of endometriosis-associated pain in teenagers. Hence, patients should be given options in selecting patients for either medical or surgical modality of treatment. Thus, GnRHa may be an effective alternative for those teenagers who have completed their bone formation.[10,11]

Progestins

Due to lack of data, usage of progestins in teenagers is of debate. This may be probably due to long-term use of progestins on bone mineral density (BMD). Some studies have shown that women who used depomedroxyprogesterone acetate (DMPA) on long term have lower BMD. Due to this reason The National Institute for Health and Care Excellence, UK (UK NICE) has recommended that care should be taken before recommending DPMA as a treatment option for adolescents. Thus, it may be an alternative option only if other methods are not suitable or not acceptable.[6]

Dienogest

Dienogest 2 mg can be started at any day of the menstrual cycle once a day, and it appears to be safe and effective when taken up to 2 years. Though, current treatments are limited to shorter treatment intervals. DNG is effective in treating symptomatic women with rectovaginal endometriosis even in a particular endometriotic subpopulation of norethisterone acetate (NETA) "resistant" patients. DNG can be a novel alternative for extragenital endometriosis.

Treatment of adolescent endometriosis with DNG is not inferior as compared to that of GnRHa. DNG was found to be successful in those patients with deep infiltrating endometriosis with or without visceral involvement; a slight reduction in BMD is noted only after 24–52 weeks of treatment (Flowchart 1).[12]

Surgery

Surgery is often indicated in those adolescent teens who have:
- Pain (failed medical management)
- Endometrioma (which damages ovary)
- Moderate or severe disease distorting anatomy
- Infertility.

Surgical options in adolescent teens will include laparoscopy rather than laparotomy. Surgery should be timed ideally in the follicular phase of her menstrual cycle, in order to prevent future possibility of recurrences and adhesions. The goal of surgical treatment is the possible removal of visible areas of endometriosis and restores their normal anatomy by adhesiolysis (Fig. 3).[13,14]

The advantages of laparoscopy are:
- Magnification
- Better visualization of subtle lesions

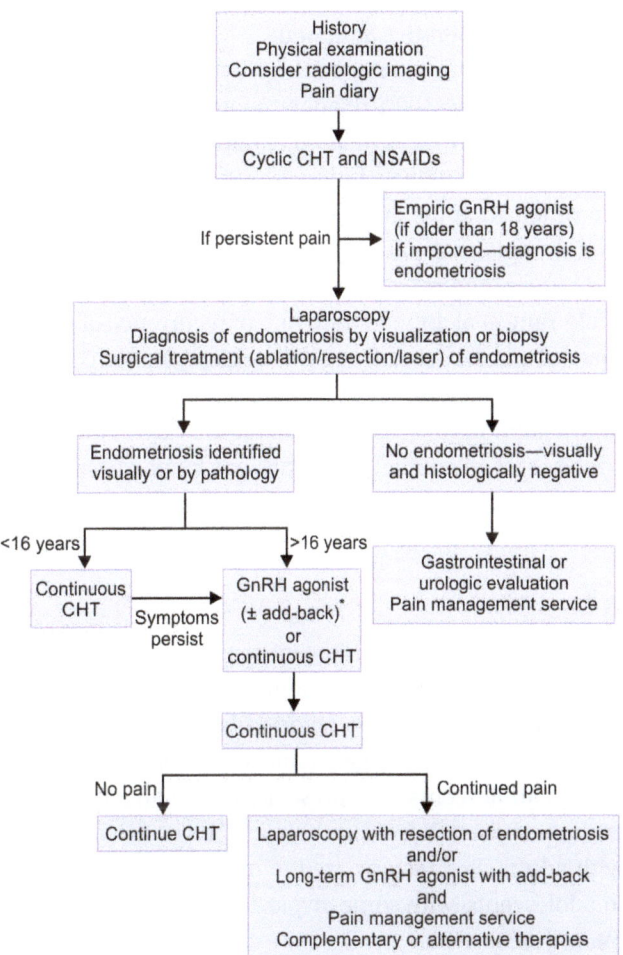

Flowchart 1: The American College of Obstetricians and Gynecologists has put forth a stepwise treatment algorithm for treatment of adolescent endometriosis.

(NSAIDs: nonsteroidal anti-inflammatory drugs; CHT: combination hormone therapy; GnRH: gonadotropin releasing hormone)
*Add-back indicates use of estrogen and progestin or norethindrone acetate alone.

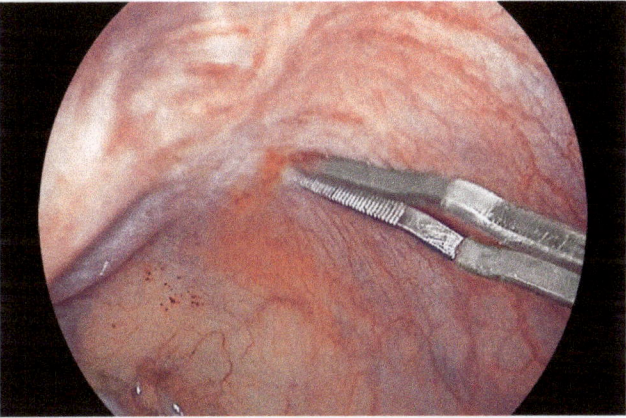

Fig. 3: Surface endometriosis electrocoagulation.
Courtesy: Rao Hospital, Coimbatore.

- Less tissue trauma and desiccation
- Smaller incisions
- Speedy postoperative recovery
- Less postoperative adhesions.

The procedure seems to improve the endometriotic symptoms in 38–100% of adolescents. Laser vaporization and monopolar or bipolar coagulation are the methods used, with no single technique shown to be superior than the other. In some studies it is reported that complete laparoscopic excision by experts can significantly reduce the recurrence rates of endometriosis in adolescents, while Yang et al. found a zero rate of recurrence of the disease (diagnosed visually or histologically) after complete laparoscopic excision of the disease in teenagers at a repeat laparoscopy for pain. Even though frequency of adolescents who undergo laparoscopy for persistent recurrent pain is 47.1%, the rate of endometriosis found at surgery was almost insignificant.[11]

ENDOMETRIAL CYSTS MANAGEMENT

Endometrioma of ovary is the most common symptomatic presentation of advanced endometriosis in adolescents. Recent publications have reported large number of cases of adolescents with stage III and IV endometriosis. Even though adolescents may present with advanced stages of endometriosis, these numbers are fewer as comparing with adults. Red lesions are the most usual lesions seen in adolescents, with some atypical lesions being common among these teens.

Ovarian endometriomas are usually correlated with more advance stage of the disease. Therefore, it is easily understood that these girls will present with more frequent pain. A retrospective study of 63 adolescents with endometrioma found bilateral disease in 22.22%, while endometrioma in the right ovary seems to be more frequent than a left endometrioma (65% vs. 57%).[13] In these cases the preferable surgery is a combined technique of cystectomy and cauterization of the capsule. Interestingly, in a review by Gordts et al. it was found that early ablative surgery can contribute to a lower morbidity, relief of symptoms, and a better quality of life, while in another recently published study have reported recurrence rates of endometrioma per patient at 24, 36, 60, and 96 months after laparoscopic cyst enucleation for ovarian endometrioma being 6.4%, 10%, 19.9%, and 30.9%, respectively. All these adolescents had stage III or IV of the disease (Figs. 4 and 5).[14]

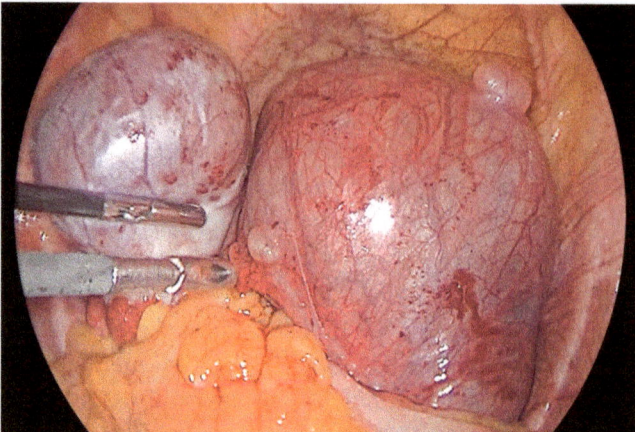

Fig. 4: Ovarian endometrioma in a 16-year-old adolescent and drainage of endometriotic cyst.
Courtesy: Rao Hospital, Coimbatore.

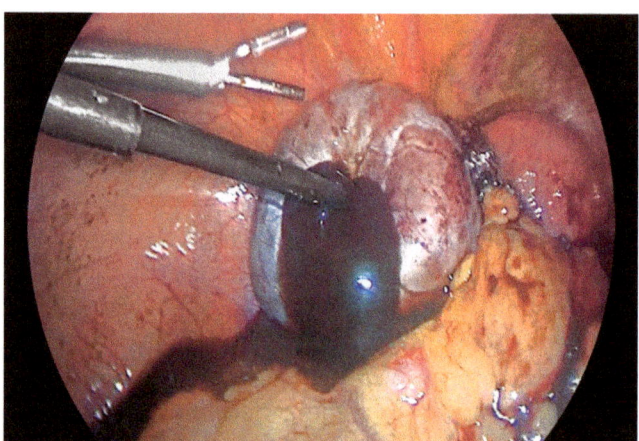

Fig. 5: Ovarian endometrioma in a 16-year-old adolescent and drainage of endometriotic cyst.
Courtesy: Rao Hospital, Coimbatore.

ROLE OF POSTOPERATIVE HORMONAL SUPPRESSION

On the other hand, postoperative hormonal suppression should be offered to adolescents in order to treat symptoms and to prevent disease progression and/or recurrence of the disease, while the role of postoperative medical therapy in addition with surgery in improving future fertility of adolescents with endometriosis has not been well documented.

However, the conjunction of surgery with postoperative medical therapy does not seem to slow disease progression and/or recurrence. The recurrence rate of endometriosis in these young women appears to be higher than in older women. In a retrospective cohort study of 57 women, aged ≤21 years, who were treated initially by excisional surgery, it was shown that the rate of recurrence of symptoms during a follow-up period of 5 years was 56%. The study also showed that the postoperative medical therapy did not influence the recurrence rates.[15]

As reported above, a variety of medical therapies have been used in treating endometriosis during adolescence. Even though further studies are needed, in order to conclude which medical therapy is superior than the other, GnRHas seem to be more effective as compared with COCs and progestins to prevent disease recurrence.

Conjugated equine estrogens as add-back therapy in combination with norethindrone acetate will be more effective for increasing total bone mineral content, BMD, and lean mass than using the usual norethindrone acetate monotherapy. LNG-IUS is accepted for use in the adolescent population for contraception and menorrhagia in sexually active women, but there are not enough data regarding its effectiveness in the treatment of adolescent endometriosis.[16]

In those studies of adults with endometriosis, *DNG* has shown limited effects on BMD. In a 24-week trial, Strowitzki et al. observed a 0.25% increase in mean lumbar spine BMD with DNG 2 mg vs. a decrease of 4.04% with leupride acetate (LA).[12]

RECURRENCE FOLLOWING SURGERY

Tandoi et al. reported that recurrence of endometrioma following surgery seems to be high during a 5-year follow-up, 56% recurrence rate has been reported among 57 young women aged ≤ 21 years. In that only 34% of these recurrences were confirmed laparoscopically and remaining 66% diagnosis of recurrence was based on either symptoms or ultrasound findings.[10] In contrast, Yeung et al. found no visual or histological evidence of recurrence in 8 of 17 teenagers (47%) who underwent repeat laparoscopy within 66 months following laparoscopic treatment of endometriosis.[17]

Majority of the studies have supported for postoperative use of medical management in order to prevent recurrence. Most of studies have reported the use of either COC pill or LNG-IUS. Now, recent studies have advocated the use of either GnRHa or DNG as an effective alternative. DNG 2 mg is equivalent in efficacy to LA for reducing endometriosis-associated pelvic pain. It is the most effective in reducing the recurrence of endometrioma, and therefore the necessity of reoperation may be avoided.[12]

There is currently no consensus whether surgery should be avoided or should be considered at an early stage. Some authors advocate conservative approach due to high recurrence rates whereas others recommend an early intervention before developing more severe lesions. Hence, further future research is required for better patient compliance.

FUTURE TRENDS

Selective estrogen receptor modulators and selective progesterone receptor modulators are the newer treatment options available for adolescent endometriosis. Both of these drugs will act by suppressing estrogen-dependent endometrial growth without any adverse systemic effects like vasomotor symptoms and loss of BMD. Another treatment options are aromatase inhibitors which are the key enzyme in estrogen biosynthesis as it appears to be overexpressed in areas of endometriosis. These drugs act by reducing ovarian and as well as local production of estrogens, and hence it can be used in treatment of adolescent endometriosis. Autoimmune modulators with antitumor necrosis factor therapies may be an effective option for disease treatment to reduce endometriotic growth in animal models, being a promising prospective future treatment model.

FOLLOW-UP

A careful follow-up of adolescents with history and symptoms of endometriosis is mandatory as it can be a life-long disease. Patients should be examined every 3–6 months for disease progression. Thus, pain calendar should be monitored, while concerns regarding future fertility and quality of life should be enrolled in the diary. Unless contraindicated, most of those patients should be put on COCs after surgery. In case if the patient has recurrence of symptoms in spite of either medical or surgical management, other treatment modalities should be considered. A multidisciplinary approach should be usually considered, including a gynecologist along with surgeon, gastroenterologist, psychologist, and urologist.

ISSUES OF INTEREST FOR FUTURE CONSIDERATION

Future studies should be ideally focused on the role of early diagnosis of endometriosis and treatment in progression and advancement of the disease process. There is a need to evaluate the course of endometriosis in teenagers, as this may improve our understanding for the development of deep endometriosis.

CONCLUSION

Due to increasing awareness of endometriosis in teenagers, increasing prevalence of the disease is being documented. Clinicians should take more proactive approach in the diagnosis and treatment of endometriosis in the teenage group. Both medical and surgical treatment options should be better utilized for them to prevent recurrence. However, a number of debatable questions are unanswered and the importance of prospective data collection/international collaboration is mandatory in order to give a better quality of care for these teens.

REFERENCES

1. ACOG Committee Opinion. Obstet Gynecol. 2018;132(6).
2. Kaur KK, Allahbadia G, Singh M. An update on diagnosis and management of adolescent endometriosis: A short communication. Acta Sci Paediat. 2019;2:48-50.
3. Deligeoroglou E, Karountzos V, Tsimaris P, et al. Endometriosis in adolescence: Challenges and opportunities for managing future infertility. Int J Gynecol Clin Pract. 2018;5:IJGCP-145.
4. ESHRE Guideline of the European Society of Human Reproduction and Embryology. 2018.
5. Brosens I, Gordts S, Benagiano G. Endometriosis in adolescents is a hidden, progressive and severe disease that deserves attention, not just compassion. Hum Reprod. 2013;28(8):2026-31.
6. Endometriosis: Diagnosis and management, NICE Guideline, 2017.
7. Miller JA, Missmer SA, Vitonis AF, et al. Prevalence of migraines in adolescents with endometriosis. Fertil Steril. 2018; 109(4):685-90.
8. Hugh S, Taylor G, Adamson D, et al. An evidence-based approach to assessing surgical versus clinical diagnosis of symptomatic endometriosis. Int J Gynecol Obstet. 2018;142:131-42.
9. Giuseppe G, Guo SW, Puttemans P, et al. Progress in the diagnosis and management of adolescent endometriosis: An opinion. Reprod Biomed Online. 2018;36(1):102-14.
10. Tandoi I, Somigliana E, Riparini J, et al. High rate of endometriosis recurrence in young women. J Pediatr Adolesc Gynecol. 2011;24(6):376-9.
11. Yang Y, Wang Y, Yang J, et al. Adolescent endometriosis in China: a retrospective analysis of 63 cases. J Pediatr Adolesc Gynecol. 2012;25:295-9.
12. Ebert AD, Dong L, Merz M, et al. Dienogest 2 mg daily in the treatment of adolescents with clinically suspected endometriosis: The VISanne Study to Assess Safety in ADOlescents. J Pediatr Adolesc Gynecol. 2017;30:560-7.
13. Gordts S, Puttemans P, Gordts S, et al. Ovarian endometrioma in the adolescent: a plea for early-stage diagnosis and full surgical treatment. Gynecol Surg. 2015;12:21-30.
14. Vitonis AF, Baer HJ, Hankinson SE, et al. A prospective study of body size during childhood and early adulthood and the incidence of endometriosis. Hum Reprod. 2010;25:1325-34.
15. Sadler GJ, Feldman HA, Stokes NA, et al. The effects of gonadotropin-releasing hormone agonist combined with add-back therapy on quality of life for adolescents with endometriosis: A randomized controlled Trial. J Pediatr Adolesc Gynecol. 2017;30:215-22.
16. Özyer S, Uzunlar Ö, Özcan N, et al. Endometriomas in adolescents and young women. J Pediatr Adolesc Gynecol. 2013;26:176-9.
17. Yeung P Jr, Sinervo K, Winer W, et al. Complete laparoscopic excision of endometriosis in teenagers: is postoperative hormonal suppression necessary? Fertil Steril. 2011; 95(6):1909-17.

CHAPTER 3

Imaging in Endometriosis

Bharti Jain, Maansi Jain

INTRODUCTION

Endometriosis is a debilitating disease of reproductive years with varied manifestations, all affecting the reproductive potential. The effect of endometriosis is multifocal. It commonly affects the pelvic organs primarily the ovaries, bowel, bladder, and peritoneum, but it can affect sites as superficial as the scar or as remote as the lung. Endometriosis is full of dilemmas for the treating doctor, both in diagnosis and treatment.[1] The common issues which arise in the diagnosis of endometriosis are its varied manifestations, lack of specific signs and symptoms, varying sensitivity and specificity of the diagnosing modalities which varies with the site involved.[2,3]

IMAGING IN ENDOMETRIOSIS

The diagnosing modalities are the ultrasonography (USG), magnetic resonance (MR), histopathology, and the operative modality, the laparoscopy.[4-7] There is absence of specific signs and symptoms of endometriosis and each diagnostic modality has its limitations in that the sensitivity and specificity varies with the site involved. Current recommendations state that for definite diagnosis of endometriosis, visual inspection at laparoscopy is the gold standard (level 3 evidence by endometriosis special interest group--ESHRE). In addition, the specificity of laparoscopy is so high that visual assessment of the disease has been accredited by the American Society for Reproductive Medicine (ASRM), the American Reproductive Society to grade the severity of endometriosis. Currently worldwide the classification system to grade the severity is being done by laparoscopy. Not only is laparoscopy the gold standard but this *see and operate modality* has a therapeutic role as well. But laparoscopy has its limitations also, as assessment of pouch of Douglas (POD) is limited in the presence of dense adhesions. Hence, deeply infiltrative disease may be underestimated in severity on laparoscopy. Also, there are limitations to diagnose posterior pelvis, bowel, and bladder disease.

The microscopic correlation, a must of nearly all pathologies is not essential to diagnose the disease. Positive histology confers the diagnosis but negative report does not exclude endometriosis. It is to be highlighted that lesions like blister lesions though pathognomonic of endometriosis may be false negative on histopathology. Visual inspection is usually adequate but histological confirmation of at least one lesion is ideal and should be done to diagnose endometriosis and exclude malignancy [good practice points (GPP)], though rare. As per ESHREE guidelines, it is controversial if histopathology should be done if only peritoneal disease is present.

As far as biochemical tests, CA-125 is usually raised in all cases of endometriosis. There have been some studies which suggest that severity/therapeutic response can be assessed by assaying CA-125. Recommendations till date by all the societies (level A) are against the practice of assaying CA-125 in endometriosis. Moreover, the patients get unduly panicked about malignancy as CA-125 rise is always raised in malignancy. Hence, the use of CA-125 should be strongly discontinued.

Ulrasonograpy and MR are the two noninvasive modalities which are being used to diagnose endometriosis and are strongly recommended. However, there are often dilemmas as to which diagnostic modality to choose. Both have their advantages and limitations. USG has high sensitivity and specificity in diagnosing ovarian endometriomas, rectal endometriosis. Transvaginal sonography (TVS) is recommended for ovarian endometrioma and transrectal ultrasound (TRUS) for rectal endometriosis (endometriosis special interest group of ESHRE). TVS also has a role in diagnosing bladder or rectum endometriosis level and TRUS for rectal lesions to diagnose or exclude endometriosis. The USG has limitations in diagnosing peritoneal implants, plaque lesions, adhesions and it has limited field of view. MR is recommended if clinical evidence of deeply infiltrative endometriosis, ureteral, bladder, bowel involvement is suspected (GPP) or to map the disease. GPP recommends that MR is not the recommended modality for endometriosis-associated infertility.

The infertility expert is most frequently concerned about ovarian endometrioma. Endometriomas are ectopic endometrial implants in the ovarian tissue which undergo cyclical hemorrhage resulting in a pseudocyst. They have varied appearances on USG. USG helps not only in diagnosing endometriomas but also in planning the patient management. The USG report should mention the morphology, size, ovarian reserve, and associated anatomical distortion. The morphology seen on USG is very pathognomonic of endometriosis. As per the International Ovarian Tumor Analysis (IOTA) classification, endometriomas are complex cysts, i.e. cysts with internal contents—residue of chronic hemorrhage but no solid content. Majority of endometriosis are unilocular, but may be multilocular—usually up to three locules. Most frequently a multilocular endometrioma is a composite mass of closely abutting separate endometriomas (Fig. 1). A classical appearance of endometrioma has a carpet of diffuse homogeneous low-level echoes, with echoes are akin to those of liver (Fig. 2). Since, it is a complex cyst, there is posterior enhancement. There are no solid areas, area of calcification, and usually no septae. But sometimes there are fibrin strands in the cyst due to superadded subacute hemorrhage. These fibrin strands are differentiated from septa as in contrast to septae fibrin strands do not traverse the wall completely and may show cyclical change. These septae should not have nodularity, solid areas. Presence of homogeneous low echoes and absence of nodularity in the wall arrows the diagnosis in favor of endometriosis. However, additional features like diffuse wall thickening with echogenic foci have been observed in endometriosis. Patel et al. have in their study seen that 20% of endometriomas had solid appearing wall or nodularity of wall, a feature predisposing/associated with malignancy.

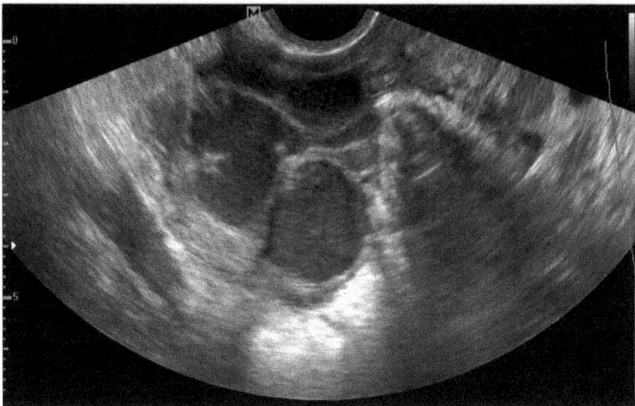

Fig. 1: Multiple endometriomas.

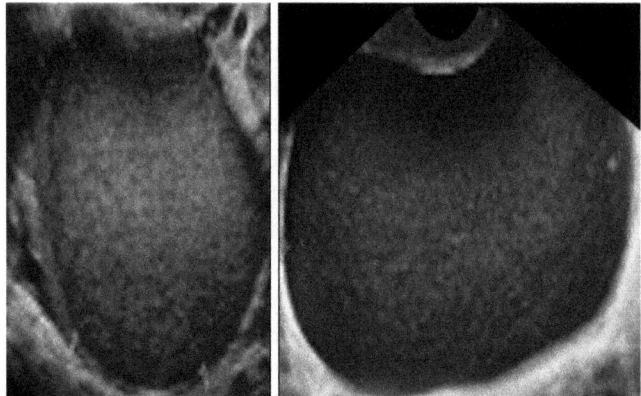

Fig. 2: Endometrioma—complex cyst with ground glass homogeneous echoes.

Sometimes superadded subacute hemorrhage may mimic a papillary lesion or solid area. They can be differentiated from solid areas as the lead edge of endometriotic lesion is not convex nor it has internal vascularity. Another feature of endometriomas is echogenic foci in the wall which is often overlooked. In a study by Patel et al., 35% of patients show echogenic foci against 6% in nonendometriomas. Echogenic foci have been postulated to correlate with cholesterol deposits resulting from repeated hemorrhage. Atypical endometrioma may present as persisting anechoic cysts, with no hormonal activity which differentiates them from functional cysts.

The differentials are hemorrhagic cyst, corpus luteal cyst as both share hemorrhage. However, both show cyclical changes and seldom show homogeneous echoes. Corpus luteal cyst has a characteristic perilesional circumferential good vascularity with low resistance flow. Other differentials are complex cysts like dermoid, serous, and mucinous cystadenoma. Dermoids have characteristic features like fat-fluid level with less echogenic fluid in the dependent part, floating fat globules, calcification, dot and dash-dermoid mesh, hyperechoic area with distal acoustic shadowing. Serous and mucinous cystadenomas are cysts—uniocular or multilocular. Cystadenomas show acoustic streaming with streaming velocities in the range 0.8–2 cm for mucinous cystadenomas and 1.5–3.6 cm for serous cystadenomas. Acoustic steaming assessment may prove to be an additional useful tool in ovarian cysts larger than 2 cm with internal echoes as in most studies endometriomas lack acoustic streaming as it is not seen in the presence of clotted blood.

Size of the lesion is crucial for management and should be mentioned. Size more than 4 cm requires surgery as per ASRM recommendations. However, the current practice with all assisted reproductive technology (ART) consultants is to avoid surgery as surgery further depletes ovarian reserve.

Repeated cyclical hemorrhage from implants in ovary causes replacement of ovarian tissue and hence depletion of ovarian reserve. So, it is imperative to assess ovarian reserve at scan by seeing D2-D3 antral follicle count. This helps to plan the management by deciding between intrauterine insemination (IUI) versus in vitro fertilization/intracytoplasmic sperm injection (IVF/ICSI) and patient counseling.

Repeated hemorrhage also causes architectural distortion and adhesions. It disturbs ovarian-uterine-tubo-peritoneal relationship—an important cause of infertility and affecting treatment plan. Hydrosalpinx caused by adhesions require corrective surgery prior to ART if seen on USG. Findings suggesting architectural distortion are kissing ovaries, sliding sign in which when gentle pressure is applied by TVS probe, anterior rectum freely glides across postaspect of cervix and postvaginal wall and rectosigmoid glides freely over posterior aspect of uterus. Absence of sliding occurs when POD is obliterated. Accuracy of this sign is around 93%.

Ultrasonography is highly sensitive and specific in diagnosing and can help plan the therapeutic approach. Hence, TVS remains the prime diagnostic modality in infertility patients.

Magnetic resonance is another noninvasive diagnostic modality of indispensable role in endometriosis. The advantage of MR—its ability to characterize hemorrhage and its age lends advantage in imaging. Also, MR offers a larger field of view, effect of adhesions on surrounding structures can be imaged.[7-9] It is better than laparoscopy in assessing involvement of POD.[9-11] In MR pulse sequences, plane of imaging is important in MR but contrast administration is not required. Chronic hemorrhage of endometriosis is hyperintense on T1W and T1FS sequences and shading on T2W sequences.[6-10] In MR adhesions are seen as spiculated low-intensity stranding which obscures organ interphases and anatomy—retroverted and displaced uterus, ovaries, angulated bowel loops, elevated postvaginal fornix, loculated fluid collection and hydrosalpinx (Fig. 3). GPP recommends that MR is not the recommended modality for endometriosis-associated infertility. There are specific indications of recommending MR in endometriosis are—when malignancy is suspected, when diagnosis is in doubt especially in virgins when TVS scan cannot be done.

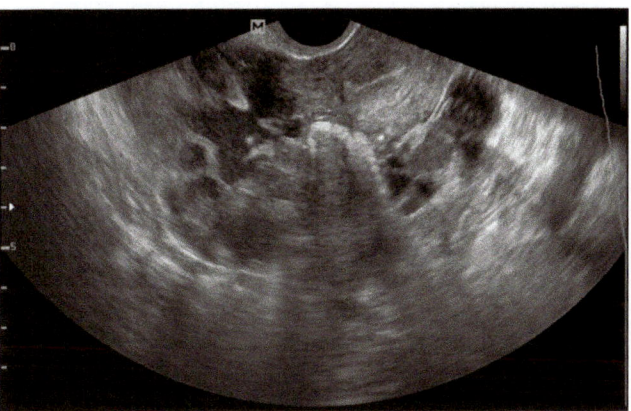

Fig. 3: Endometriomas with adhered bowel.

CONCLUSION

Good Practice Points (GPP) recommends that TVS is indispensable in diagnosis of endometriosis especially ovarian involvement and planning the management of infertility. MR is not the recommended modality for endometriosis-associated infertility.

REFERENCES

1. Practice bulletin no. 114: Management of endometriosis. Obstet Gynecol. 2010;116(1):223-36.
2. Chapron C, Dubuisson JB, Pansini V, et al. Routine clinical examination is not sufficient for diagnosing and locating deeply infiltrating endometriosis. J Am Assoc Gynecol Laparosc. 2002;9(2):115-19.
3. Clement PB. The pathology of endometriosis: a survey of the many faces of a common disease emphasizing diagnostic pitfalls and unusual and newly appreciated aspects. Adv Anat Pathol. 2007;14(4):241-60.

4. Bazot M, Thomassin I, Hourani R, et al. Diagnostic accuracy of transvaginal sonography for deep pelvic endometriosis. Ultrasound Obstet Gynecol. 2004;24(2):180-5.
5. Bazot M, Lafont C, Rouzier R, et al. Diagnostic accuracy of physical examination, transvaginal sonography, rectal endoscopic sonography, and magnetic resonance imaging to diagnose deep infiltrating endometriosis. Fertil Steril. 2009;92(6):1825-33.
6. Bazot M, Darai E, Hourani R, et al. Deep pelvic endometriosis: MR imaging for diagnosis and prediction of extension of disease. Radiology. 2004;232(2):379-89.
7. Abrão MS, Gonçalves MO, Dias JA Jr, et al. Comparison between clinical examination, transvaginal sonography and magnetic resonance imaging for the diagnosis of deep endometriosis. Hum Reprod. 2007;22(12):3092-97.
8. Chamié LP, Blasbalg R, Gonçalves MO, et al. Accuracy of magnetic resonance imaging for diagnosis and preoperative assessment of deeply infiltrating endometriosis. Int J Gynaecol Obstet. 2009;106(3):198-201.
9. Gonçalves MO, Dias JA Jr, Podgaec S, et al. Transvaginal ultrasound for diagnosis of deeply infiltrating endometriosis. Int J Gynaecol Obstet. 2009;104(2):156-60.
10. Kinkel K, Chapron C, Balleyguier C, et al. Magnetic resonance imaging characteristics of deep endometriosis. Hum Reprod. 1999;14(4):1080-6.
11. Chapron C, Vieira M, Chopin N, et al. Accuracy of rectal endoscopic ultrasonography and magnetic resonance imaging in the diagnosis of rectal involvement for patients presenting with deeply infiltrating endometriosis. Ultrasound Obstet Gynecol. 2004;24 (2):175-79.

CHAPTER 4

Medical Management of Endometriosis and Adenomyosis—What's New

Sonia Malik, Meenakshi Dua

INTRODUCTION

Endometriosis is a chronic medical disorder characterized by the presence of endometrial glands and stroma outside the endometrial cavity. There are very few studies from India however, the general incidence is quoted in the Federation of Obstetric and Gynecological Societies of India (FOGSI) good clinical practice recommendations (GCPR) 2016, as 10% of the women of reproductive age group. Among the infertile women 25–48% suffers from endometriosis. 176 million women or even more in the world suffer from endometriosis.[1]

Endometriosis has been a challenging medical condition for the treating physician and very debilitating for the patients. It is a diagnostic dilemma for physicians with majority of patients being asymptomatic or presenting with atypical symptoms. The final diagnosis requires laparoscopy and histopathology of the lesions, which further delays the management. It presents with two major problems pain and infertility. All medical therapies are therefore directed at managing these two symptoms. All the currently available therapies are having a contraceptive effect since they target anovulation for the suppression of endometriosis hence, are unsuitable for those requiring fertility. However, medical therapy in such patients is indicated when they are awaiting surgery or antiretroviral therapy (ART) or for long-term suppression in order to avoid another surgery when treatment has failed.

Adenomyosis is a common benign gynecological disorder, akin to endometriosis, characterized by the presence of endometrial glands and stroma within the myometrium. The pathophysiology is nearly similar but restricted to the uterus. Hence, treatment currently is similar to that of endometriosis and will be described together in this text.

MEDICAL MANAGEMENT OF ENDOMETRIOSIS

In recent years, a lot of research has gone into the development of new therapies for the treatment of endometriosis. Most currently available therapies target the underlying biochemical abnormalities and the therapeutic targets. Some of the critical underlying mechanisms that lead to the symptoms of endometriosis are:[2]
- Exaggerated inflammatory responses
- Excess production of estrogen, and
- Progesterone resistance.

Studies have shown that the endometriotic implants have impaired molecular and immunological functions. This leads to increased production of estrogen, proinflammatory cytokines, prostaglandins, and metalloproteinases and a failure of immune cells to suppress and clear the inflammatory response.

Estrogen is crucial for the growth and persistence of the endometriotic implants, which comes from various sources.
- The endometrial implants have intrinsic aromatase activity, which leads to the conversion of cholesterol to estradiol.[3]
- The endometrium is rich in prostaglandin E2 (PGE2) receptors and activation of the PG receptor subtype EP-2 leads to activation of cyclic AMP, which increases the expression of key steroidogenic genes, and aromatase activity eventually leading to increased estradiol production.
- Along with intrinsic aromatase activity estradiol produced from ovary and peripheral fat also reaches the sites of endometriosis.

This continuous supply of estrogen is important for the continuous growth and survival of endometriotic implants.

> **BOX 1:** Pathophysiology of endometriosis.
> - Increases production of estradiol
> - Increased intrinsic aromatase activity
> - Increased production of inflammatory markers
> - Progesterone resistance

Pelvic pain in endometriosis is secondary to increased concentrations of PGs especially of the subtype E2 and F2α.[4] This increased concentration of PGE2 also provides a stimulus for estrogen production. Studies have shown that along with estradiol and PGE2, there is a role of cytokines, especially IL-1β and angiogenic factors like vascular endothelial growth factor (VEGF) in inducing cyclo-oxygenase-2 (COX2) expression and increased PG production in endometriotic implants.

Growing evidence also now suggests a role of progesterone resistance in endometriosis (Box 1). Studies have shown that the endometriotic lesions have a low progesterone receptor level.[5] Progesterone is important for the activation of key enzyme 17-beta-hydroxy-steroid-dehydrogenase 2, which helps in converting estradiol to estrone, which is less biologically active. Thus increased production of estradiol and decreased clearance leads to the growth of the endometriotic tissue.[6]

ENDOMETRIOSIS AND MEDICATIONS

The medical management of endometriosis is targeted toward controlling pain and suppression of the hormonally active endometriotic tissue. Over the years, several therapeutic options have been developed and successfully used to achieve these aims and newer targets are also being developed at a fast pace. While a trial of nonsteroidal anti-inflammatory drugs (NSAIDs) as first-line therapy can be helpful in controlling the pain, hormonal therapies that cause suppression of the endometriotic tissues, e.g. combined oral contraceptives, progesterone only contraceptives, gonadotropin-releasing hormone (GnRH) agonists, aromatase inhibitors, and danazol can be used for long-term treatment (Box 2).

Nonsteroidal Anti-inflammatory Drugs

Nonsteroidal anti-inflammatory drugs are the most commonly used first-line agents in the management of endometriosis related pain and dysmenorrhea. The pain in endometriosis is mostly secondary to elevated levels of PGs, interleukins and cytokines. NSAIDs work by blocking the enzyme COX that is crucial for the production of the

> **BOX 2:** Medications used in endometriosis.
>
> *Hormonal*:
> - Combined oral contraceptives
> - Progesterone containing contraceptives:
>   - Oral or injectable
>   - Implant
>   - Levonorgestrel-containing intrauterine system (LNG-IUS)
> - Selective progesterone receptor modulators:
>   - Mifepristone
>   - Ulipristal acetate
>   - Onapristone
> - Gonadotropin-releasing hormone agonists:
>   - Leuprolide acetate
>   - Nafarelin
>   - Goserelin
> - Gonadotropin-releasing hormone antagonists:
>   - Cetrorelix
>
> *Nonhormonal*:
> - NSAIDs
> - Aromatase inhibitors
> - Danazol

(NSAIDs: nonsteroidal anti-inflammatory drugs)

inflammatory mediators. Although, both COX1 and COX2 receptors are present, studies have shown that the ectopic endometrial tissues have a higher concentration of COX2 receptors. Along with pain control, new studies have shown that selective COX2 inhibitors like rofecoxib can also inhibit the growth of the endometrial tissue.[7] Despite inconclusive evidence regarding effectiveness of NSAIDs in controlling endometriosis related pain and negative gastrointestinal side effect profile, a trial of NSAIDs is the most common first intervention in patients with pelvic pain.

Combined Hormonal Contraceptives

The suppression of ovaries and disease activity forms the basis of the use of hormonal contraceptives in endometriosis and they are the most commonly used first-line hormonal therapy. Estrogen and progesterone combinations or progesterone alone lead to decidualization of the endometriotic tissue and slows the progression of the disease. They have been used with varying degree of success in women with endometriosis. Cost, ease of administration, and tolerability are some of the advantages that have led to their popularity. Continuous therapy with combined oral contraceptive (COC) has been shown to have better pain control as compared to cyclic administration.[8] However, the limiting factors include long-term administration, risk of thromboembolism, high rates of recurrence after discontinuation and impaired fertility due to contraceptive action. Combinations containing lower dose of ethinyl estradiol (20 μg) as compared to high dose (30 μg) have a lower risk of venous thromboembolism and are currently recommended.[9]

Gonadotropin-releasing Hormone Agonists

The use of GnRH agonists is based on the fact that it leads to profound hypoestrogenism by blocking ovarian estrogen production and hence regression of endometriotic implants. There is initially a flare effect with the release of follicle-stimulating hormone (FSH) and luteinizing hormone (LH); however, chronic administration leads to downregulation of pituitary GnRH receptors that results in suppression of the hypothalamic pituitary ovarian axis leading to anovulation. This eventually leads to hypoestrogenism, amenorrhea and regression of the endometriotic implants by depriving the implants of estrogen that is crucial for their survival. This is a good option for women who have failed initial therapy with oral contraceptive pills (OCPs) or are not candidates for OCPs due to their medical history. GnRH agonists are available in both nasal and injectable forms and offer high rates of pain relief and longer symptom free period for up to 12 months.[10] Leuprolide acetate 3.75 mg monthly injection or 11.25 mg used three monthly, goserelin and nafarelin are the most commonly used preparation. However, they are approved for continuous use for only up to 6 months due to concerns of side effects secondary to hypoestrogenism like bone loss, vaginal atrophy and dryness, hot flashes and abnormalities in lipid profile.[11] The addition of add-back therapy provides symptomatic relief and decreases the rate of bone loss. Another limitation of the use of GnRH agonists is that they suppress ovulation and cannot be used in women desiring fertility.

Gonadotropin-releasing Hormone Antagonists

These are another group of drugs that have shown promising results in the treatment of endometriosis. Compared to GnRH agonists they do not cause the initial flare and have lower degree of hypoestrogenism and a better side effect profile with equivalent symptomatic improvement. In their study, Kupker et al. showed that administration of GnRH antagonist cetrorelix provided symptomatic relief and regression of the endometriotic implants as visualized on laparoscopy.[12] With a lower degree of hypoestrogenemia and better tolerance than the GnRH agonists they offer a great potential in the treatment of endometriosis.

Progesterone-containing Contraceptives

Progesterone has multiple mechanisms of action that form the pathophysiologic basis of its use in endometriosis. It induces decidualization of the endometrium, inhibits estrogen induced mitosis, alters estrogen receptors, and inhibits angiogenesis and expression of matrix metalloproteinase needed for the growth of the endometriotic implants.[13,14] Available in different forms oral, injectable or intrauterine device, they have gained popularity and are a great option for women with contraindications to estrogens. Some of the progestins that have been studies and used in the treatment of endometriosis include cyproterone acetate, dienogest, dydrogesterone, gestrinone, lynesterole, medroxyprogesterone acetate, megestrol acetate, and norethindrone acetate.

Medroxyprogesterone is available as oral and injectable preparation and can be administered 150 mg intramuscularly every 3 months. Although, there is no standardized oral dose, studies using different doses of oral medroxyprogesterone from 10 mg/day to 100 mg/day for 3–6 months have reported varying degree of improvement in endometriosis related pain.[15,16] Injectable progesterone offers the added advantage of better compliance by avoiding daily administration and erratic gastrointestinal absorption.

Dienogest, a 19-nortestosterone derivative, is another progestin that has been studied in the treatment of endometriosis. It has high specificity for progesterone receptors and less anti-androgenic side effects. Continuous administration leads to decidualization and atrophy of the endometrial lesions. It also has anti-inflammatory, antiangiogenic and antiproliferative effects. In a dose of 2 mg or 4 mg/day, dienogest has been shown to have a favorable profile for safety and efficacy; patients reported improvement in the endometriosis related symptoms and an overall improvement in quality of life.[17,18] It is in general well tolerated and side effects included irregular bleeding, which improves with time.

Levonorgestrel-containing Intrauterine Systems

Levonorgestrel-containing intrauterine system is a T-shaped device that contains 52 mg of levonorgestrel, which releases 20 micrograms of hormone per day over a 5-year period. Multiple studies have shown the efficacy of levonorgestrel-containg intrauterine system (LNG-IUS) in women with endometriosis due to progesterone induced atrophy of the endometrium and higher concentration of progesterone in the peritoneal cavity suppressing the activity of ectopic endometrium by anti-inflammatory and immunomodulatory functions.[19] There are also reports of successful use in patients with adenomyosis and deep rectovaginal endometriosis.[20] In another study comparing LNG-IUS to depot administration of GnRH analogs, similar efficacy was reported with lower incidence of hypoestrogenic side effects in women using the intrauterine device.[21] With its long-term use and better side effect profile LNG-IUS offers a great option in women who do not desire to conceive.[22] More research is underway to understand the long-term efficacy in women with endometriosis.

Etonogestrel Implant

Another route of progesterone delivery that has been studied is the subdermal implant also commonly known as implanon. Inserted intradermally in the arm, it contains progestin etonogestrel and offers contraceptive benefits for 3 years. The improvement in dysmenorrhea seen in women using it for contraception prompted research for its use in endometriosis. Walch et al. in their study compared the therapeutic efficacy of depot medroxyprogesterone acetate and implanon in 41 women with endometriosis and reported that both groups had similar incidence of pain relief and both groups had similar side effect profile and degree of satisfaction.[23] Commonly reported side effects include irregular menstrual bleeding, weight gain, nausea, headache, breast tenderness, acne that are similar to depot medroxyprogesterone acetate. In carefully selected women who do not desire fertility etonogestrel implant could be another option for symptomatic endometriosis.

Selective Progesterone Receptor Modulators

Selective progesterone receptor modulators (SPRMs) are a relatively new class of agents that have tissue effect ranging from pure agonists to agonist/antagonist to antagonist. Mifepristone and ulipristal acetate are the two SPRMs that are commonly used. Mifepristone, which has a predominant progesterone antagonist effect, has been used for medical abortions and ulipristal acetate for emergency contraception. Selective inhibition of endometrial growth without the side effects of hypoestrogenism, decreased menstrual bleeding via effect on the endometrial blood supply and suppression of endometrial blood supply are some of the mechanisms that have prompted their use in endometriosis. In animal models, treatment with ulipristal acetate has shown to result in atrophy of the endometrium and suppression of estrogen dependent endometrial growth.[24,25] Decreased expression of COX-2 has also been shown in rat models treated with mifepristone and ulipristal acetate.[26] Studies in humans are however limited. In one study, Kettel et al. studied nine women with endometriosis treated with mifepristone 50 mg/day for 6 months and all nine women reported an improvement in pelvic pain without significant side effects of hypoestrogenism.[27]

Aromatase Inhibitors

Aromatase enzyme helps in the conversion of the steroid precursors into estrogen. The ovaries and the fat are the predominant source of the enzyme but other sources include skin, placenta and the brain. Studies have shown that aromatase over expressed in endometriosis.[28] Aromatase induced estrogen synthesis leads to the growth of the endometrial implants, COX expression, prostaglandin secretion, which further induces aromatase activity. Unlike GnRH agonists, aromatase inhibitors block estrogen synthesis both in the periphery and the ovaries. This mechanism is particularly helpful in postmenopausal women with endometriosis where peripheral fat is the predominant source of estrogen. Anastrozole, letrozole, and exemestane are third generation aromatase inhibitors that can be administered orally. They are reversible, more potent and have faster onset of action. Used in combination with combined oral contraceptives, GnRH agonists or progesterone, they significantly decrease the endometriosis-associated pain, improve quality of life and have shown to decrease the size of the lesion. However, their side effects include ovarian follicular cyst and bone loss with long-term use. Oral contraceptives and progestins if prescribed as add back therapy can decrease the bone loss.

Danazol

Danazol, a derivative of 17 alpha-ethinyl-testosterone, is an androgenic agent that inhibits LH surge and decreases ovarian steroidogenesis by direct inhibition of the ovarian enzymes. Usually given in divided doses of 400–800 mg/day for 6 months. Side effects include acne, hirsutism, deepening of voice, weight gain, muscle cramps, liver dysfunction and an abnormal lipid profile. A meta-analysis by Selak et al. showed that when treated with danazol, patients had improved laparoscopic scores and decreased pain symptoms as compared to placebo or no treatment.[29] However, adverse effects related to hyperandrogenism limit their use. As the side effects are mostly associated with oral administration, alternative routes of like danazol vaginal ring and intrauterine devices are currently in research and studies have shown improvement in pain symptoms with better tolerability.[30,31]

FUTURE THERAPIES

Endometriosis is a disease of reproductive age women. It is bound to grow with each menstruation. So, during this period patient needs to be continuously on medical therapy for its suppression. These medical therapies create a pseudomenopausal state thus affecting fertility of these patients. This warrants search for new molecules/drugs which can suppress endometriosis without affecting fertility.

Antiangiogenesis Factors

Endometriotic lesions grow by forming network of capillaries around them and this helps in the growth and survival of the lesions. Studies have also shown that these lesions secrete angiogenic factors like VEGF and the peritoneal fluid is rich in angiogenic factors. In theory, halting the growth of new blood vessels could stop the growth of new lesions and regresses older ones.

Dopamine receptor 2 agonists, cabergoline and quinagolide have been shown to reduce angiogenesis by dephosphorylation of VEGF2. They have been used safely in humans for the treatment of hyper-prolactinemia and lactation suppression. They have been found to be successful in reducing size of endometriotic lesion in mice.[32] In a human study, Gomez et al. studied 9 women with endometriosis-associated hyperprolactinemia, women first had a surgical procedure where half of the endometriotic lesions were excised and the other half was marked. This was followed by treatment with quinagolide for 18–20 weeks followed by a second laparoscopy. They showed a significant reduction in the size of the lesion and down regulation of VEGF/VEGF2, proangiogenic cytokines and plasminogen activator inhibitor (PAI-1).[33]

Various anti-angiogenic factors are being tried in the treatment of endometriosis. However, these agents are still in early development with most of the research on animal models. Agents like TNP-470 (an analogue of antibiotic fumagilin), endostatin (a proteolytic fragment of collagen with endogenous anti-angiogenic activity), anginex (a synthetic peptide that stops the growth of blood vessels and induces apoptosis), and anti-VEGF antibody (Avastin) have been successful in decreasing the size of endometriotic lesions in animal models; however, no data is available in humans.

Statins

Statins are cholesterol lowering drugs and have been used for decades for hypercholesterolemia. It has anti-inflammatory, antiangiogenic and antioxidant properties.[34] Atorvastatin, simvastatin, mevastatin and lovastatin have in animal models. Sharma et al reported an increased inhibition of inflammatory and angiogenic genes (COX-2, VEGF, RAGE, and EN-RAGE) in atorvastatin treated endometrial-endometriotic cells. They also reported increased expression of anti-inflammatory genes (PPAR-γ and LXRα and IGFBP-1).[35] Similarly, in another study, simvastatin is found to reduce size and number of endometriotic lesions in mouse model by reducing matrix metalloproteinase.[36] However, human trials are needed for same.

Tumor Necrosis Factor α Blockers

Endometriosis is associated with inflammation. Degree of inflammation varies with grade of endometriosis. Tumor necrosis factor α (TNFα) is a proinflammatory cytokine which is found to be raised in endometriosis. TNFα blockers are have been successfully used in the treatment of inflammatory conditions like rheumatoid arthritis and Crohn's disease. Infliximab, a monoclonal antibody against TNFα and etanercept, a fusion protein with the ability to neutralize TNFα are being actively studied in the treatment of endometriosis. These have shown benefits in animal models.[37] More human trials are needed for its support.

Pentoxifylline

Lately pentoxifylline has been found to have TNFα blocking properties in animal trials.[38] It was successful in improving fertility and size of endometriotic lesions. However, recent meta-analysis in humans did not show any reduction in size of lesions or improvement in clinical pregnancy rates in women treated with pentoxyphylline.[39]

CONCLUSION

In short, endometriosis is an enigmatic disease. It is a chronic illness with frequent recurrences requiring prolonged treatment. Surgery gives good results but does not cure it and cannot be offered at every relapse. Medical therapy helps in not just preventing relapse but also, in treating microlesions left behind postsurgery. As it affects women of reproductive age group, most of the times it is associated with fertility issues. Choice of treatment should be based on complaint of patient. Patients with infertility should be offered surgery/short term medical therapy followed by ART. Most of the currently used medical therapy affects fertility and hence cannot be used for long term in these women. Prolonged medical therapy benefits fertile women postsurgery for prevention of relapse, women with chronic pelvic pain or women with menorrhagia due to adenomyosis/endometriosis.

REFERENCES

1. Bendigeri T, Warty N, Sawant R, et al. Endometriosis: Clinical Experience of 500 Patients from India. Indian Pract. 2015; 68(7):34-40.
2. Bulun SE. Endometriosis. N Engl J Med. 2009;360(3):268-79.
3. Zhao H, Zhou L, Shangguan AJ, et al. Aromatase expression and regulation in breast and endometrial cancer. J Mol Endocrinol. 2016;57(1):R19-33.
4. Jabbour HN, Sales KJ, Smith OP, et al. Prostaglandin receptors are mediators of vascular function in endometrial pathologies. Mol Cell Endocrinol. 2006;252(1-2):191-200.
5. Attia GR, Zeitoun K, Edwards D, et al. Progesterone receptor isoform A but not B is expressed in endometriosis. J Clin Endocrinol Metab. 2000;85(8):2897-902.
6. Bulun SE, Cheng YH, Yin P, et al. Progesterone resistance in endometriosis: link to failure to metabolize estradiol. Mol Cell Endocrinol. 2006;248(1-2):94-103.
7. Dogan E, Saygili U, Posaci C, et al. Regression of endometrial explants in rats treated with the cyclooxygenase-2 inhibitor rofecoxib. Fertil Steril. 2004;82(Suppl 3):1115-20.
8. Zorbas KA, Economopoulos KP, Vlahos NF. Continuous versus cyclic oral contraceptives for the treatment of endometriosis: a systematic review. Arch Gynecol Obstet. 2015;292(1):37-43.
9. Lidegaard O, Nielsen LH, Skovlund CW, et al. Risk of venous thromboembolism from use of oral contraceptives containing different progestogens and oestrogen doses: Danish cohort study, 2001-9. BMJ. 2011;343:d6423.
10. Winkel CA, Scialli AR. Medical and surgical therapies for pain associated with endometriosis. J Womens Health Gend Based Med. 2001;10(2):137-62.
11. Prentice A, Deary AJ, Goldbeck-Wood S, et al. Gonadotrophin-releasing hormone analogues for pain associated with endometriosis. Cochrane Database Syst Rev. 2000;(2):CD000346.
12. Kupker W, Felberbaum RE, Krapp M, et al. Use of GnRH antagonists in the treatment of endometriosis. Reprod Biomed Online. 2002;5(1):12-16.
13. Whitehead MI, Townsend PT, Pryse-Davies J, et al. Effects of various types and dosages of progestogens on the postmenopausal endometrium. J Reprod Med. 1982;27 (Suppl 8):539-48.
14. Bruner KL, Eisenberg E, Gorstein F, et al. Progesterone and transforming growth factor-beta coordinately regulate suppression of endometrial matrix metalloproteinases in a model of experimental endometriosis. Steroids. 1999;64(9):648-53.
15. Moghissi KS, Boyce CR. Management of endometriosis with oral medroxyprogesterone acetate. Obstet Gynecol. 1976;47(3):265-7.
16. Luciano AA, Turksoy RN, Carleo J. Evaluation of oral medroxyprogesterone acetate in the treatment of endometriosis. Obstet Gynecol. 1988;72(3 Pt 1):323-7.
17. Schindler AE. Dienogest in long-term treatment of endometriosis. Int J Womens Health. 2011;3:175-84.
18. Köhler G, Faustmann TA, Gerlinger C, et al. A dose-ranging study to determine the efficacy and safety of 1, 2, and 4mg of dienogest daily for endometriosis. Int J Gynaecol Obstet. 2010;108(1):21-5.
19. Vercellini P, Vigano P, Somigliana E. The role of the levonorgestrel-releasing intrauterine device in the management of symptomatic endometriosis. Curr Opin Obstet Gynecol. 2005;17(4):359-65.
20. Fedele L, Bianchi S, Zanconato G, et al. Use of a levonorgestrel-releasing intrauterine device in the treatment of rectovaginal endometriosis. Fertil Steril. 2001;75(3):485-8.
21. Petta CA, Ferriani RA, Abrao MS, et al. Randomized clinical trial of a levonorgestrel-releasing intrauterine system and a depot GnRH analogue for the treatment of chronic pelvic pain in women with endometriosis. Hum Reprod. 2005;20(7):1993-8.
22. Vercellini P, Frontino G, De Giorgi O, et al. Comparison of a levonorgestrel-releasing intrauterine device versus expectant management after conservative surgery for symptomatic endometriosis: a pilot study. Fertil Steril. 2003;80(2):305-9.
23. Walch K, Unfried G, Huber J, et al. Implanon versus medroxyprogesterone acetate: effects on pain scores in patients with symptomatic endometriosis—a pilot study. Contraception. 2009;79(1):29-34.
24. Gopalkrishnan K, Katkam RR, Sachdeva G, et al. Effects of an antiprogestin onapristone on the endometrium of bonnet monkeys: morphometric and ultrastructural studies. Biol Reprod. 2003;68(6):1959-67.
25. Brenner RM, Slayden OD, Nath A, et al. Intrauterine administration of CDB-2914 (Ulipristal) suppresses the endometrium of rhesus macaques. Contraception. 2010;81(4):336-42.
26. Huniadi CA, Pop OL, Antal TA, et al. The effects of ulipristal on Bax/Bcl-2, cytochrome c, Ki-67 and cyclooxygenase-2 expression in a rat model with surgically induced endometriosis. Eur J Obstet Gynecol Reprod Biol. 2013; 169(2):360-5.
27. Kettel LM, Murphy AA, Morales AJ, et al. Treatment of endometriosis with the antiprogesterone mifepristone (RU486). Fertil Steril. 1996;65(1):23-8.
28. Bulun SE, Zeitoun KM, Takayama K, et al. Molecular basis for treating endometriosis with aromatase inhibitors. Hum Reprod Update. 2000;6(5):413-8.

29. Selak V, Farquhar C, Prentice A, et al. Danazol for pelvic pain associated with endometriosis. Cochrane Database Syst Rev. 2007;4:CD000068.
30. Igarashi M, Iizuka M, Abe Y, et al. Novel vaginal danazol ring therapy for pelvic endometriosis, in particular deeply infiltrating endometriosis. Hum Reprod. 1998;13(7):1952-6.
31. Igarashi M, Abe Y, Fukuda M, et al. Novel conservative medical therapy for uterine adenomyosis with a danazol-loaded intrauterine device. Fertil Steril. 2000;74(2):412-3.
32. Delgado-Rosas F, Gomez R, Ferrero H, et al. The effects of ergot and non-ergot-derived dopamine agonists in an experimental mouse model of endometriosis. Reproduction. 2011;142(5):745-55.
33. Gomez R, Abad A, Delgado F, et al. Effects of hyperprolactinemia treatment with the dopamine agonist quinagolide on endometriotic lesions in patients with endometriosis-associated hyperprolactinemia. Fertil Steril. 2011;95(3):882-8 e881.
34. Yilmaz B, Ozat M, Kilic S, et al. Atorvastatin causes regression of endometriotic implants in a rat model. Reprod Biomed Online. 2010;20(2):291-9.
35. Sharma I, Dhawan V, Mahajan N, et al. In vitro effects of atorvastatin on lipopolysaccharide-induced gene expression in endometriotic stromal cells. Fertil Steril. 2010; 94(5): 1639-46 e1.
36. Bruner-Tran KL, Osteen KG, Duleba AJ. Simvastatin protects against the development of endometriosis in a nude mouse model. J Clin Endocrinol Metab. 2009;94(7):2489-94.
37. Cayci T, Akgul EO, Kurt YG, et al. The levels of nitric oxide and asymmetric dimethylarginine in the rat endometriosis model. J Obstet Gynaecol Res. 2011;37(8):1041-7.
38. Perello M, Gonzalez-Foruria I, Castillo P, et al. Oral Administration of Pentoxifylline Reduces Endometriosis-Like Lesions in a Nude Mouse Model. Reprod Sci. 2017; 24(6):911-918.
39. Song H, Lu D, Li Y, et al. Pentoxifylline for endometriosis. Cochrane Database Syst Rev. 2012;1:CD007677.

CHAPTER 5

Adenomyosis and Assisted Reproductive Technology

Kuldeep Jain, Maansi Jain, Bharti Jain

INTRODUCTION

Adenomyosis is an emerging enigmatic disease for the clinicians, particularly the assisted reproductive technology (ART) consultants. It is associated with dilemmas and gray areas in almost all aspects—be it epidemiology, diagnosis or treatment. Initially it was diagnosed only in parous women with the definitive diagnosis made on specimens obtained after hysterectomy on histology. Currently with better imaging techniques, it is being diagnosed with increasing frequency at earlier age and in patients with subfertility in infertility clinics. The dilemmas for clinicians begin with determining the accuracy of diagnostic tests to help screen adenomyosis early and setting gold standards of universally acceptability. Another area is to study the impact on infertility and the need for treatment of adenomyosis. Also, the efficacy of medical versus surgical fertility-sparing treatment needs further elucidation as also the reproductive and obstetric outcome in adenomyosis with or without treatment.

EPIDEMIOLOGY

Initially, adenomyosis was considered a disease of parous women over 40 years, however it is now being diagnosed with increasing frequency in younger nulliparous women at infertility clinics. But a casual association between adenomyosis and subfertility is not fully established as of date with some advocating that adenomyosis is infrequent in subfertile women, while others incriminating adenomyosis in subfertility:[1]
- Affects 30% of young women
- More common in Asians and Africans
- Coexist with other comorbidities like fibroids, endometriosis.

PATHOGENESIS

Adenomyosis is characterized by disruption of the normal boundary between the endometrial basal layer and the myometrium with consequent benign invasion of endometrial glands into the myometrium. This ectopic adenomyotic foci should be at least 2.5 cm away from junctional zone to differentiate it from minimally invaginated basal endometrium. This innate endometrium gives rise to ectopic intramyometrial glands that cause reactive hypertrophy and hyperplasia of adjacent myometrium.[2] Postulated hypothesis is endometrium invaginating in the myometrium with facilitation by hyperestrogenism and mechanical forces causing dysperistalsis. Functional eutopic endometrium with its innate properties compounded by altered smooth muscles of myometrium are speculated to be incriminated. Evidence pointing causal association to endometrial invagination along intramyometrium lymphatics is weak as it can explain only stromal myosis but fails to explain presence of functioning glands. Some proponents speculate influence of steroids in the pathogenesis. They point to local rather than systemic hyperestrogenism. There is a higher E2 in menstrual but not peripheral blood via aromatase on androgen precursors conversion of estrone-3-sulp to estrone by estrone sulfatase. In secretory phase, there is increased conversion of E2 to estrone because of altered 17-B hydrosteroid dehydrogenase type-2. Also, in adenomyosis stromal and endometrial cells have a distinct proteomic profile. Also some endometrial cells have some features of smooth muscles resembling fibroblasts in proliferative phase and immature cells in secretory phase.

This suggests some plasticity in endometrial myometrial interphase. Some suggest altered angiogenesis as evidenced by polymorphism of two angiogenic factors, fibroblasts growth factor 1 and 2.

DIAGNOSIS

Reference standard for adenomyosis is histopathology. On histopathology in adenomyosis, there is the presence of ectopic endometrium in the myometrium. However, different definitions vary in terms of the distance of eutopic endometrial foci from the endometrial myometrial junction. Some define this minimum distance as one low power field (×10) others define it as one medium (×100) or high-power field and in some it is 2.5 mm as a minimal distance in the diagnostic criteria of adenomyosis. This threshold distance needs to be defined to differentiate it from minimal invagination of basal endometrium which is a physiological variant.

Ultrasonography (USG) parameters used to define adenomyosis are—heterogeneous myometrial area, globular asymmetric enlarged uterus with asymmetrical anterior or posterior wall, nonhomogeneous myometrial echoes, irregular cystic spaces, myometrial linear striations, poor definition of endometrial myometrial junction (Figs. 1 to 3). But there is no consensus on the number of parameters required for diagnosis. Vercellini et al. (1998) used only one parameter,[3] while some recommend the presence of all parameters for diagnosis.[4]

Magnetic resonance imaging (MRI) is considered as the gold standard among noninvasive diagnostic tools. But there is a need to define threshold criteria and have internationally agreed definitions with defined cut-off thresholds for thickness of junction zone, the prime diagnostic criteria.[5] Some use expansion of anterior and posterior junctional zone (without mentioning any specific thickness), on the other hand some use a junctional zone thickness of >9, Kissler et al. (2008),[1,6] some set this thickness threshold to 12 mm. Other features of adenomyosis on MRI are a large, asymmetric uterus without leiomyomas, ill-defined junctional zone, low-signal intensity myometrium in contrast to well-circumscribed mass in fibroid, punctuate high-intensity myometrial foci.

EFFECT OF ADENOMYOSIS ON INFERTILITY

Better imaging techniques enabled earlier detection of adenomyosis on USG and MRI in nulliparous females

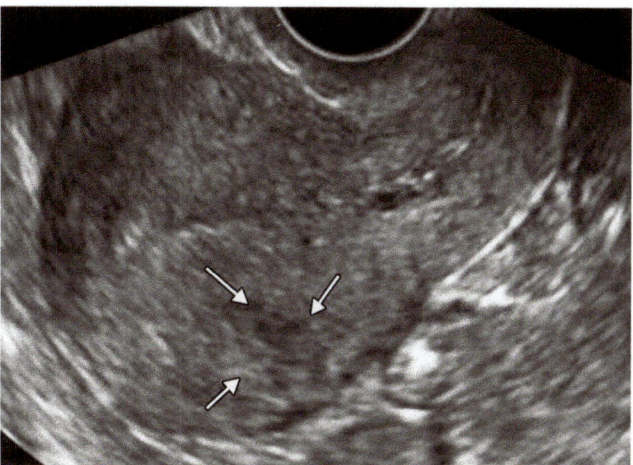

Fig. 1: Focal adenomyosis.

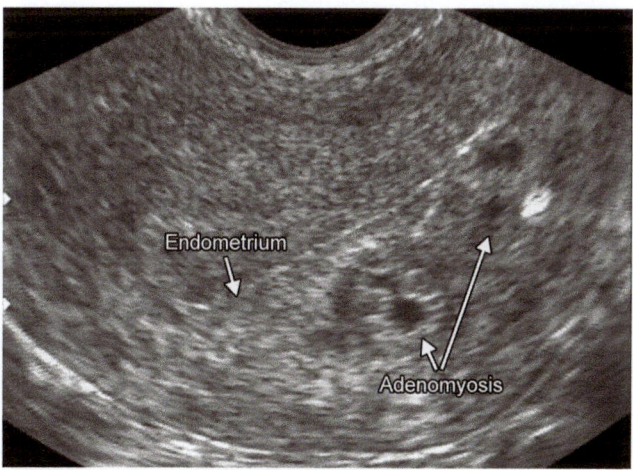

Fig. 2: Myometrial cysts.

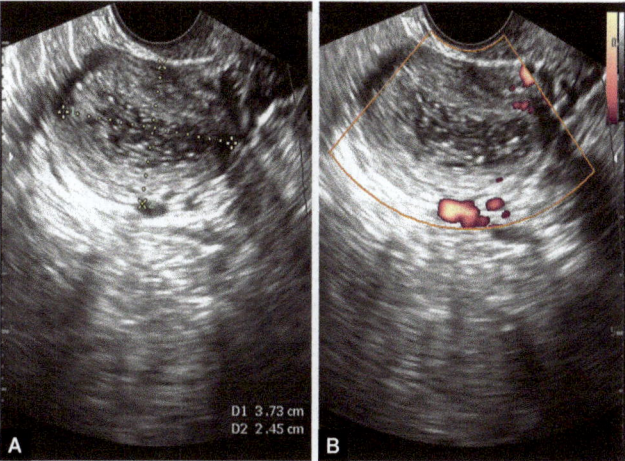

Figs. 3A and B: Unusual presentation large focal adenomyosis with collection of blood.

attending infertility clinics. So, this change in the trend toward detecting adenomyosis at an earlier age in nulliparous infertile females from the earlier trend which labels adenomyosis as a disease prevalent in the fourth or fifth decade leads to the speculation whether adenomyosis is the cause of infertility. This question becomes more imperative in unexplained infertility when there is no cause seen. So, emerged the dilemma for the clinicians whether adenomyosis is associated with infertility and if so, is treatment required. On literature search no study was found which aimed to see the effect of adenomyosis on fertility in natural cycles. Main impedance in pregnancy was speculated to be implantation failure esp. in ART cycles.[6,7] Martínez-Conejero et al. (2011) also document increased miscarriage rate/implantation failure in adenomyosis.[8] But on the other hand two conflicting studies show no effect of adenomyosis.[9,10]

Tremellen and Russell (2011)[8] presented case series of 4 females with multiple IVF failure—repeated implantation failure (RIF) in which down regulation with ultralong protocol improved pregnancy rate. In contrast Mijatovic (2010) in a randomized controlled trial (RCT) of 74 women with adenomyosis associated with endometriosis showed no difference in outcome compared with 151 patients with only endometriosis in ultralong protocol.[9]

■ MEDICAL MANAGEMENT

In adenomyosis, the role of medical treatment is palliative only. The therapeutic gain is symptomatic relief and not the resorption of lesion as there is no cytoreduction. The pathology persists despite treatment with any pharmaceutical drug, irrespective of any length of treatment or any dose and the disease presents again on discontinuation.

The main challenge is in the field of infertility as the treatment is achieved by suppressing hypothalamic pituitary gonadal axis, by suppressing ovulation, abolition of mensuration, inducing a stable steroid hormonal milieu, reducing endogenous estrogen, or inducing endometrial differentiation. So gonadotropic agonists, oral contraceptive pill (OCP), progestins, selective estrogen receptor modulator (SERM), selective progesterone receptor modulator (SPRM), and aromatase inhibitors are used.

A hypoestrogenic environment [gonadotropin-releasing hormone (GnRH) agonists, AI], hyperandrogenic (danazol) or hyperprogestogenic (OCP, progestanins) is induced on treatment rendering the ectopic endometrium nonfunctional and suppressing endometrial cell proliferation.

GnRH Agonist Therapy

Spontaneous pregnancies are documented within 2 years of cessation of long-term use of GnRHa.[11] The combination therapy of conservative surgery with a GnRH agonist also has been recommended. The therapeutic advantages/preferences of GnRH agonists over conservative surgery or over GnRH agonists combined with conservative surgery are debatable and recommendations and guidelines are required in this aspect.

Combination of Conservative Surgery with GnRH Agonist/Danazol

A meta-analysis identified eight studies (4 case series and 4 case reports) evaluating conservative surgery with or without GnRH agonist. The pooled live birth rate after this mode of treatment was 88.2% (15 of 17). In six studies GnRH agonists were used and in two Danazol was used. There was a considerable heterogeneity in the type of GnRH agonist, the duration and timing of use as well as the mode of diagnosis of adenomyosis before treatment was offered.[12] A retrospective study comparing conservative surgery with GnRH agonist versus GnRH agonist alone showed live birth rates following conservative surgery versus GnRH agonist alone were 32.14% versus 8%, respectively.[13]

Other conservative treatments include high-intensity focused USG, uterine artery embolization. The use of a danazol-loaded intrauterine device or a vaginal ring in infertility patients with adenomyosis was evaluated by Igarashi et al. and they achieved a combined pregnancy rate of 41% (16 of 39) after insertion and removal of these devices.[14]

Scant data are available on uterine artery embolization and high-intensity focused USG to cause thermocoagulation are other conservative alternatives of indeterminate significance in treating infertility.

Kim et al. (2005)[15] published a study evaluating the effectiveness of uterine artery embolization in the management of adenomyosis and reported a live birth rate of 83.3% (five of six patients). Rabinovici et al. (2006)[16] published first successful live birth following USG thermos coagulation in a patient with adenomyosis.

The definitive treatment of adenomyosis is radical surgical treatment hysterectomy which is curative. This is done when multiparous female presents with dysmenorrhea, menorrhagia in the fourth or fifth decade. But when infertility is the concern, role of fertility-sparing conservative surgery for adenomyosis is debatable as it is not possible to isolate and hence excise the adenomatous tissue adequately. The reason for it is that the pathology is diffuse with indistinct boundaries with the normal tissue. Avoiding entering the uterine cavity requires skill and in 30% of cases is entered inadvertently and requires repair. Tensile strength of scar is compromised because of contained adenomyotic foci.

So, fertility-sparing surgery is done keeping this limitation in mind with the aim to improve reproductive outcome. No detrimental effect has been observed till date because of conservative fertility-enhancing surgery.

Role of conservative uterine conserving surgery compared with GNRH agonists is not clear. There are no clear indications of which and when patient should undergo fertility conserving surgery and not GnRH agonist.

It is to be noted that when the size of uterus exceeds 12 cm (>12 weeks), bulk reduction surgery should be advised followed by GnRH agonist and ART, if it fails other alternative is hysterectomy with surrogacy and it should be done/advised.

In focal adenomyosis/diffuse adenomyosis, surgery can be done by laparoscopy/or laparotomy or lap with laparotomy (Fig. 4). Laparotomy offers an advantage as palpation helps discern pathological tissue from normal. Takeuchi et al. (2006)[17] reported live birth and Strizhakov and Davydov (1995)[18] reported pregnancy after conservative surgery involving excision of the adenomyotic tissue followed by hysteroplasty either laparoscopically or via laparotomy.

An overall live birth rate of 36.2% (21 of 58) was achieved following the conservative surgery. Fujishita et al. (2004) in a retrospective study compared the classical method of adenomyomectomy with a new modified reduction surgery (transverse H incision technique). The classical technique involved a uterine incision followed by step-wise resection of adenomyotic tissue and closure. The newer technique modified the incision to the shape of an H and this was followed by raising serosal flaps and excision of the adenomyomatous tissue. The new technique was associated with a 50% pregnancy rate, compared with no pregnancy with the older classical method. The odd of having a live birth with the old classical method compared with the newer technique was 0.14 [95% confidence interval (CI), 0.00 and 4.47].[19]

The time to pregnancy was 4 and 6 months. The classical surgery involves V-shaped uterine incision followed by step-wise wedge resection of adenomyotic tissue followed by closure. Here adenomyotic tissue remains on both sides of the incision. The created wound is sutured but in the modified technique an H-shaped incision followed by raising serosal flaps and excision of the adenomyomatous tissue is done.

Another technique involves wedge-shaped removal of adenomyotic tissue with a thin margin after an incision. Another adenomyotic skill involves complete excision with a triple flap method.

Asymmetric dissection of uterus longitudinally, dissecting myometrium diagonally, opening uterine cavity transversally adenomyotic tissue excised >5 mm of inner myometrium, then >5 mm of serosal myometrium and then suturing the cavity and removal of adenomyoma by morcellator. Literature is scant when fertility-preserving surgery is making it difficult to draw conclusions.

CONCLUSION

Adenomyosis presents a challenge as there has been changes in concepts involving this disease. Now, it is detected in earlier age group in nulliparous infertile women in contrast to the previous belief that it is a disease of parous women.

Equally debatable is whether it is the cause of infertility especially unexplained infertility when there is no cause apparent for infertility. However, there is enough evidence to suggest that implantation rates, pregnancy rate, and live birth rates are significantly less in adenomyosis and high risk of miscarriage rates are reported. ideal approach for these patients is GnRH agonist followed by ART or a combination of GnRHa along with bulk reduction surgery followed by ART to give best outcome.

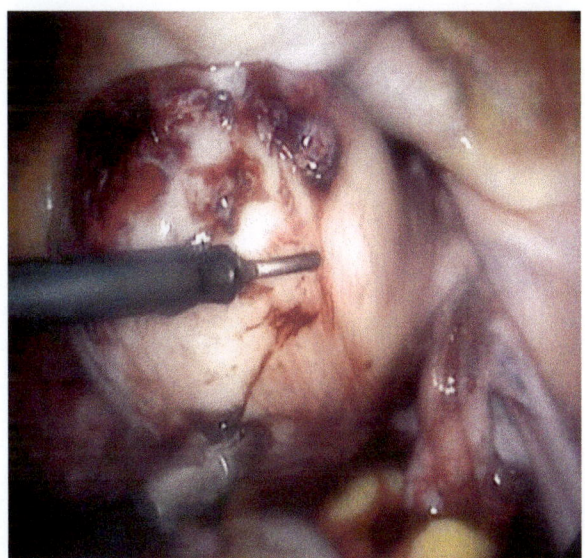

Fig. 4: Laparoscopic adenomyomectomy—large adenomyoma.

REFERENCES

1. Kissler S, Zangos S, Koh J, et al. Duration of dysmenorrhoea and extent of adenomyosis visualised by magnetic resonance imaging. Eur J Obstet Gynecol Reprod Biol. 2008;37:204-9.
2. Vercellini P, Vigano P, Somigliana E, et al. Adenomyosis: Epidemiological factors. Clin Obstet Gynaecol. 2006;20:465-77.
3. Vercellini P, Cortesi I, Giorgi O, et al. Transvaginal ultrasonography versus uterine needle biopsy in the diagnosis of diffuse adenomyosis. Hum Reprod Update. 1998;13:2884-87.
4. Sun YL, Lin P, Wang CB, et al. Transvaginal sonographic criteria for the diagnosis of adenomyosis. Taiwan J Obstet Gynecol. 2010;49:40-4.
5. Kunz G, Beil D, Huppert P, et al. Adenomyosis in endometriosis—prevalence and impact on fertility. Evidence from magnetic resonance imaging. Hum Reprod. 2005;20:2309-16.
6. Maubon A, Faury A, Kapella M, et al. Uterine junctional zone at magnetic resonance imaging: A predictor of in vitro fertilization implantation failure. J Obstet Gynaecol Res. 2010;36:611-8.
7. Tremellen K, Russell P. Adenomyosis is a potential cause of recurrent implantation failure during IVF treatment. Aust N Z J Obstet Gynaecol. 2011;51(3):280-3.
8. Martínez-Conejero JA, Morgan M, Montesinos M, et al. Adenomyosis does not affect implantation, but is associated with miscarriage in patients undergoing oocyte donation. Fertil Steril. 2011;96:943-50.
9. Mijatovic V, Florijn E, Halim N, et al. Adenomyosis has no adverse effects on IVF/ICSI outcomes in women with endometriosis treated with long-term pituitary down-regulation before IVF/ICSI. Eur J Obstet Gynecol Reprod Biol. 2010;151(1):62-5.
10. Costello MF, Lindsay K, McNally G. The effect of adenomyosis on in vitro fertilisation and intra-cytoplasmic sperm injection treatment outcome. EJOG. 2011;158(2):229-34.
11. Lin J, Sun C, Zheng H. Gonadotropin-releasing hormone agonists and laparoscopy in the treatment of adenomyosis with infertility. Chin Med J. 2000;113:442-5.
12. Maheshwari A, Gurunath S, Fatima F, et al. Adenomyosis and subfertility: A systematic review of prevalence, diagnosis, treatment, and fertility outcomes. Hum Reprod Update. 2012;18(4):374-92.
13. Wang PH, Fuh JL, Chao HT, et al. Is the surgical approach beneficial to subfertile women with symptomatic extensive adenomyosis. Obstet Gynecol. 2009;35:495-502.
14. Igarashi M, Abe Y, Fukuda M. Novel conservation medical therapy for uterine adenomyosis with a danazol-loaded intrauterine device. Fertil Steril. 2000;74:412-3.
15. Kim MD, Won JW, Lee DY, et al. Uterine artery embolisation for adenomyosis without fibroids. Clin Radiol. 2004;59:520-6.
16. Rabinovici J, Inbar Y, Eylon SC. Pregnancy and live birth after focused ultrasound surgery for symptomatic focal adenomyosis: Case report. Hum Reprod. 2006;21:1255-9.\
17. Takeuchi H, Kitade M, Kikuchi I, et al. Laparoscopic adenomyomectomy and hysteroplasty. J Minim Invasive Gynecol. 2006;13:150-54.
18. Strizhakov AN, Davydov AI. Myometrectomy—a method of choice for the therapy of adenomyosis patients in the reproductive period. Akush Ginekol (Mosk).1995;5:31-3.
19. Fujishita A, Masuzaki H, Khan KN, et al. Modified reduction surgery for adenomyosis. Gynecol Obstet Invest. 2004;57:132-8.

CHAPTER 6

Müllerian Anomalies and Endometriosis

T Ramani Devi, Dhivya Sethuraman

INTRODUCTION

Müllerian duct anomalies (MDAs) are due to incomplete development, abnormal vertical or lateral fusion, or absorption of the Müllerian ducts. The range of Müllerian anomalies includes uterovaginal agenesis, hypoplasia, unicornuate uterus, uterus didelphys, bicornuate uterus, septate uterus, and arcuate uterus (Table 1).[1]

Endometriosis is known to be associated with Müllerian anomalies. The incidence of endometriosis among Müllerian anomalies varies between 30% and 40%.[2,3] Obstructive anomalies are associated more with endometriosis, as compared to nonobstructive anomalies and this contributes, the proof in favor of theories of retrograde menstruation and coelomic metaplasia.[4]

Table 1: Classification of Müllerian anomalies (ESHRE/ESGE).

	Female genital tract anomalies				
	Uterine anomaly			Cervical/vaginal anomaly	
	Main class	Subclass		Coexistent class	
U0	Normal uterus			C0	Normal cervix
U1	Dysmorphic uterus	a. T-shaped b. Infantilis c. Others		C1	Septate cervix
				C2	Double "normal" cervix
U2	Septate uterus	a. Partial b. Complete		C3	Unilateral cervical aplasia
				C4	Cervical aplasia
U3	Bicorporeal uterus	a. Partial b. Complete c. Bicorporeal septate		V0	Normal vagina
				V1	Longitudinal nonobstructing vaginal septum
U4	Hemiuterus	a. With rudimentary cavity (communicating or not horn) b. Without rudimentary cavity (horn without cavity/no horn)		V2	Longitudinal obstructing vaginal septum
U5	Aplastic	a. With rudimentary cavity (bi- or unilateral horn) b. Without rudimentary cavity (bi- or unilateral uterine remnants/aplasia)		V3	Transverse vaginal septum and/or imperforate hymen
				V4	Vaginal aplasia
U6	Unclassified malformations				
U			C		V

(ESGE: European Society of Gastrointestinal Endoscopy, ESHRE: European Society of Human Reproduction and Embryology)

GENETIC BASIS

Abnormalities in reproductive tract development can be caused by *HOX* gene mutations or altered *HOX* gene expression. Diethylstilbestrol (DES) and other endocrine disruptors cause Müllerian defects by changing *HOX* gene expression. Alteration of *HOXA10* and *HOXA11* expression is also identified as a mechanism of decreased implantation associated with endometriosis.[5]

Women with the N314D mutation of galactose-1-phosphate uridyltransferase (GALT) are reported to have an association with vaginal agenesis. These patients showed a higher incidence of endometriosis, especially advanced disease.[6]

PREVALENCE OF MÜLLERIAN ANOMALIES

The prevalence of Müllerian anomalies varies between 7% and 9.8%.[7,8] The prevalence increases to 18% in women with recurrent pregnancy loss.[7] Arcuate and septate uterus are the most common uterine anomalies (Fig. 1).

Müllerian anomalies are more frequent in nulliparous women. Women with polycystic ovaries have a higher incidence of Müllerian anomalies, especially septate uterus.[9]

Renal agenesis is found to be associated with uterine anomalies (in almost one-third of the cases) especially in uterus didelphys, uterine agenesis, and unicornuate uterus.[10]

ENDOMETRIOSIS AND OBSTRUCTIVE MÜLLERIAN ANOMALIES

Approximately 40% of cases of obstructive Müllerian anomalies have endometriosis.[2] This is explained by retrograde menstruation theory.

One case series suggests that obstructed hemivagina, ipsilateral renal agenesis syndrome (OHVIRA syndrome) is the most common obstructive Müllerian anomaly diagnosed in adolescents after menarche.[11]

The transverse vaginal septum is a much rarer type of obstructive condition (1/2,100-1/72,000), most commonly (40%) occurring in the upper third of the vagina.[12] Segmental forms of vaginal agenesis also occur in 15% of cases and this is usually referred to as complete or partial vaginal atresia (lower vaginal atresia).[13] If the uterus is normally developed and the cervix is not present or not open to the vagina, it is termed as cervical agenesis or dysgenesis which is a rare diagnosis.

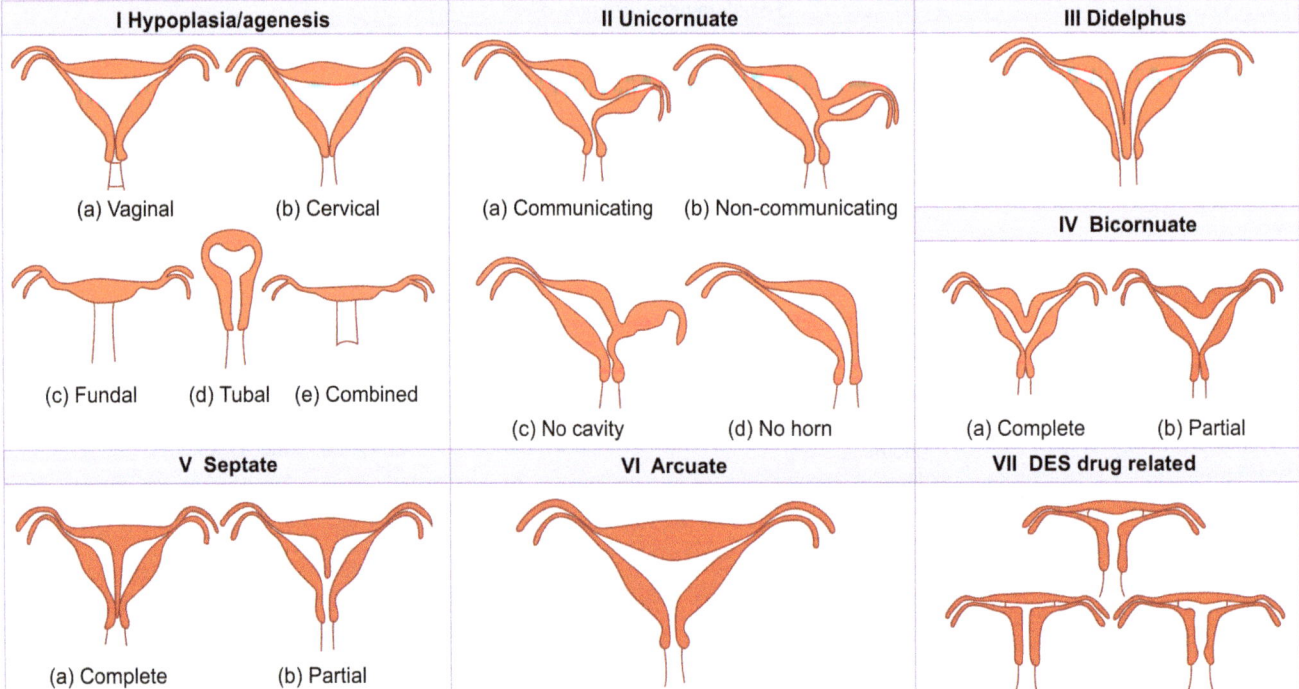

Fig. 1: ASRM classification of Müllerian anomalies (ASRM: American Society for Reproductive Medicine; DES: diethylstilbestrol).

Other Müllerian anomaly associated with endometriosis is noncommunicating uterine horn.[14] These women usually manifest with progressive severe dysmenorrhea and abdominal pain. They become symptomatic in the second decade of life.[15] Another case report describes a functioning rudimentary horn presenting as an inguinal hernia.[16]

ENDOMETRIOSIS AND NONOBSTRUCTIVE UTERINE ANOMALIES

Women with nonobstructive uterine anomalies are also at a higher risk for endometriosis. The frequency of endometriosis was found to be 30.8% in women with nonobstructive Müllerian anomalies, the prevalence being significantly greater in women with unicornuate uterus (55%).

Women with septate uterus have 26% incidence of endometriosis.[17] Such women are also prone for advanced disease.[18] A possible higher association of septate uterus with endometriosis cannot be explained by retrograde menstruation. Uterine dysperistalsis is suggested to be the mechanical cause of endometriosis in such patients.[19]

CLINICAL FEATURES

Obstructive defects are generally diagnosed in puberty, during the 1st year after the expected menstruation should have occurred and hence establishment of pubertal timeline is very important.[13]

They usually present with cyclical pain and primary amenorrhea. If not evaluated, the pain becomes severe necessitating evaluation in the emergency department.[20] An abdominal mass may be palpable in such patients secondary to hematocolpos or hematocolpometra. A bulge may be felt during the rectal examination. Sometimes acute retention of urine may be the presenting symptom.

Adolescents may also present with progressive dysmenorrhea and regular or irregular periods in the setting of an obstructed hemivagina with complete duplication of the uterine horns and upper vagina.[21] On physical examination, an abdominal mass may be palpated, if the obstruction is chronic. On examination the external genitalia are normal. A bulge is appreciated during rectal examination.

DIAGNOSIS

Usually the first imaging modality is ultrasonography. A transabdominal ultrasonography is an appropriate initial imaging modality. Rarely translabial ultrasonography can help to delineate an obstruction.[22]

Traditionally magnetic resonance imaging (MRI) is considered as the gold standard for precise diagnosis of the anomaly, to assess the depth of the vagina, the thickness of a septum, and the extent of the distension of vagina, cervix, and uterus or tubes.[23] More recently three-dimensional (3D) ultrasonography has been used, due to the cost and patients convenience when compared to MRI. The diagnostic accuracy of MRI in endometriosis depends upon the size, location, and morphology of endometriotic implants with sensitivity being least for peritoneal implants.[24]

In patients with Müllerian anomalies there is a high incidence of renal (40%) and spinal (10–20%) abnormalities. It is important to use additional imaging to screen for these problems depending on the underlying diagnosis. This can be accomplished by renal ultrasonography or MRI of the abdomen and spine.[23]

MEDICAL TREATMENT

Patients with obstructive Müllerian malformations with functional endometrium can be preoperatively managed with continuous combined low-dose monophasic oral contraceptives which cause amenorrhea to control pain and treat endometriosis. This may permit a delay in surgical intervention to facilitate other investigations and to allow thorough counseling of the patient and her family about the implications of the diagnosis.[25] Alternatively, oral progestogens, gonadotropin-releasing hormone agonist injections with add-back therapy or depot medroxyprogesterone acetate injections can also be used. Patients should be counseled that medical management is only temporary and surgery is a must.

SURGICAL TREATMENT

The definitive treatment is always surgery. Early surgical repair of the obstruction usually prevents endometriosis. For those with established endometriosis, surgery offers symptomatic relief and improves fertility.

Vaginal septa can be tackled from below, facilitating the drainage of a hematocolpos or hematometra, and aiding repair.

Laparoscopy has been an important tool for the treatment of uterovaginal anomalies. It is used to detect the anomaly, reconstruct an absent vagina, and resect abnormal Müllerian structures.[26]

Combined hysterolaparoscopy is done in patients with nonobstructive anomalies associated with endometriosis, especially septate uterus, as it allows correct diagnosis and treatment simultaneously (septostomy and excision of the endometriotic tissue).

However, endometriosis does not always resolve following repair of an obstructive anomaly. This may result from prior or ongoing peritoneal seeding or other factors. This may necessitate medical therapy or surgery in future.[27]

SYNDROMES AND ENDOMETRIOSIS

Mayer-Rokitansky-Küster-Hauser Syndrome

Mayer-Rokitansky-Küster-Hauser (MRKH) syndrome is characterized by Müllerian agenesis. Rarely these patients may show a prevalence of uterine remnants which may possess functional endometrium. Such patients will present with pelvic pain due to endometriosis.[28] The incidence of endometriosis is significantly increased in patients with unilateral rudimentary uteri.[29] These patients should be offered MRI and subsequent medical and surgical therapy.

Herlyn-Werner-Wunderlich Syndrome or OHVIRA Syndrome (Figs. 2 to 6)[30]

It is characterized by a triad of symptoms—uterus didelphys, obstructed hemivagina, ipsilateral renal agenesis, and endometrioma. It can be classified based on complete or incomplete obstructed hemivagina. The most common presentation is dysmenorrhea, chronic pelvic pain, and lower abdominal mass, secondary to hematocolpos with or without hematometra and hematosalpinx.[31] Endometriosis occurs due to retrograde menstruation. MRI is used for detailing the anatomical abnormality. Early surgical intervention relieves symptoms and prevents endometriosis.

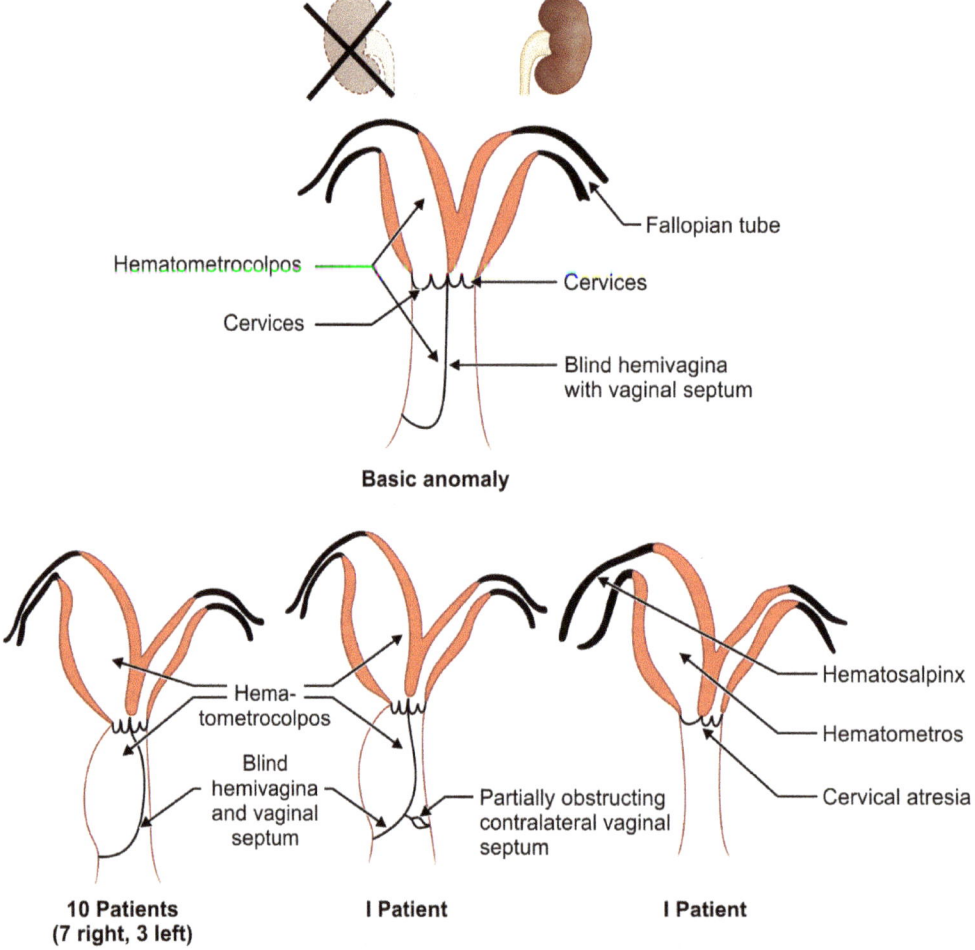

Figs. 2A and B: Schematic diagram of Herlyn-Werner-Wunderlich (HWW) syndrome.

Müllerian Anomalies and Endometriosis

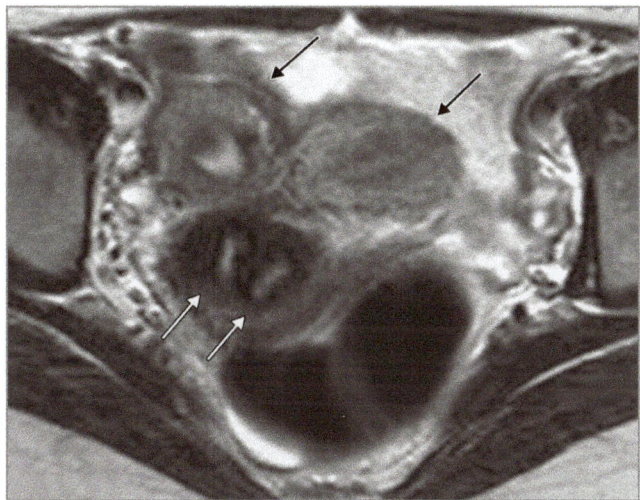

Fig. 3: Magnetic resonance imaging of Herlyn-Werner-Wunderlich (HWW) syndrome 1. White arrows indicate uterine didelphys and black arrows indicate hematometra of right horn of uterus and right ovarian endometrioma.

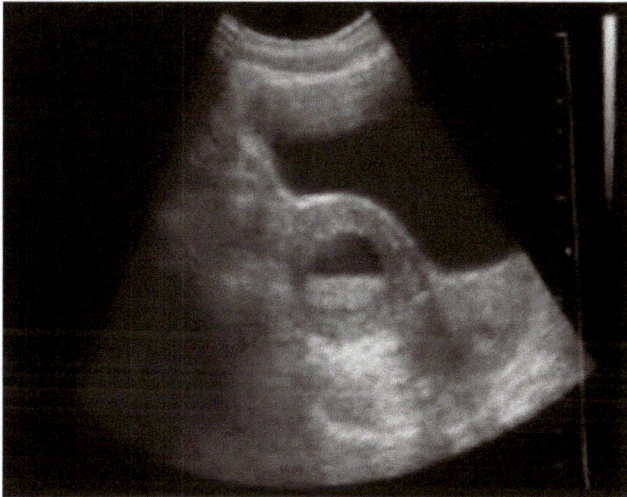

Fig. 5: Ultrasonography of hematometra of the noncanalized horn.

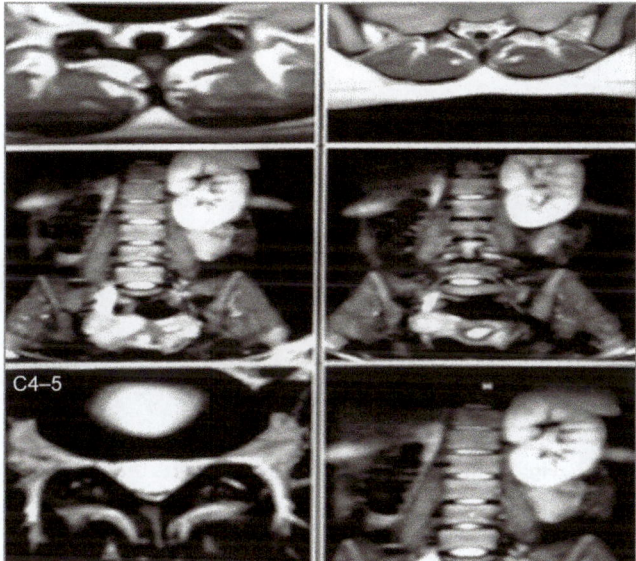

Fig. 4: Magnetic resonance imaging of Herlyn-Werner-Wunderlich (HWW) syndrome 2.

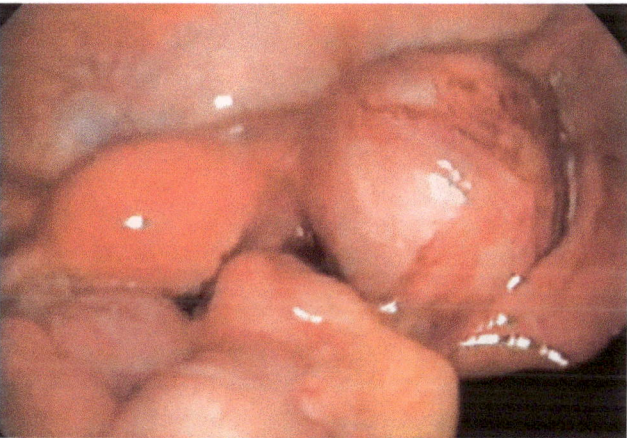

Fig. 6: Laparoscopic view of hematometra of the noncanalized horn.

Robert's Uterus (Figs. 7 to 12)[32]

Robert's uterus is a very rare Müllerian anomaly. This is characterized by the presence of atypical septum where the lower end is attached to the lateral wall instead of entering the cervix. This will lead to hematometra in the noncommunicating horn and leads to endometrioma on the same side. This can be treated by hysterolaparoscopy and septostomy, where the noncommunicating horn can be opened in to the communicating horn. Rarely horn can be excised through laparoscopy.

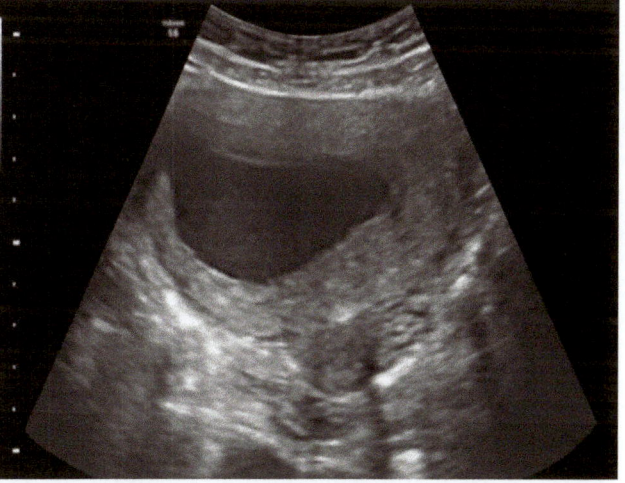

Fig. 7: Ultrasonography of Robert's uterus.

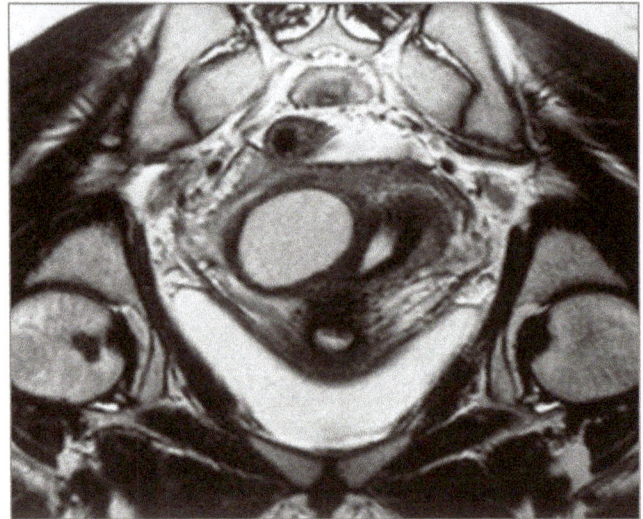

Fig. 8: Magnetic resonance imaging of Robert's uterus.

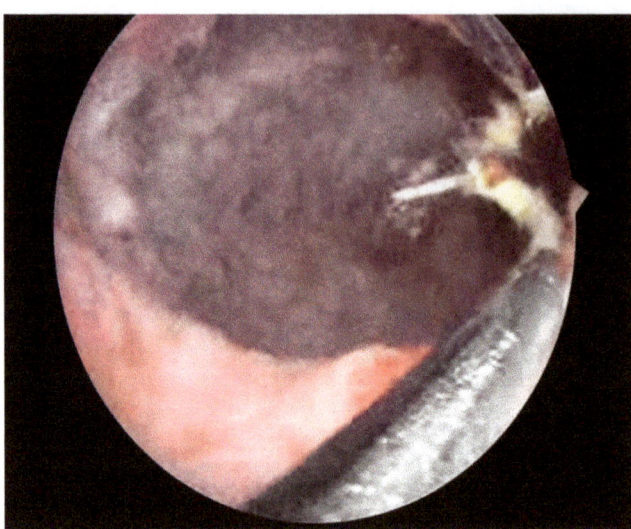

Fig. 11: Hysteroscopic resection of Robert's uterus.

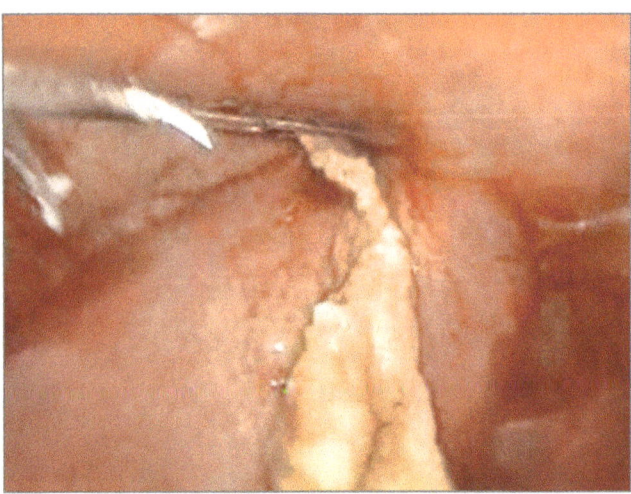

Fig. 9: Laparoscopic view of Robert's uterus.

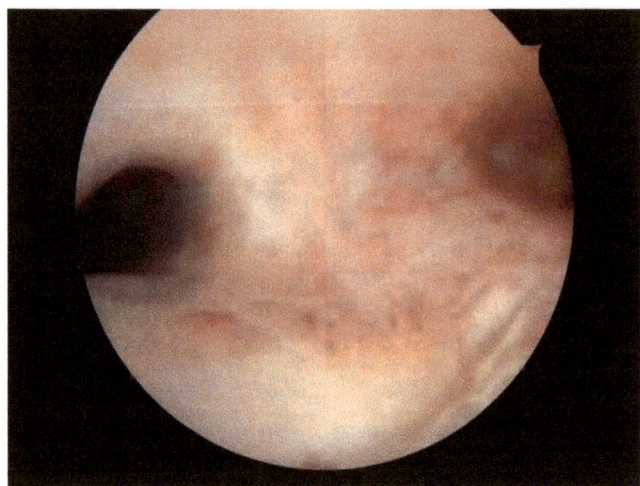

Fig. 12: Relook hysterscopic view of Robert's Uterus.

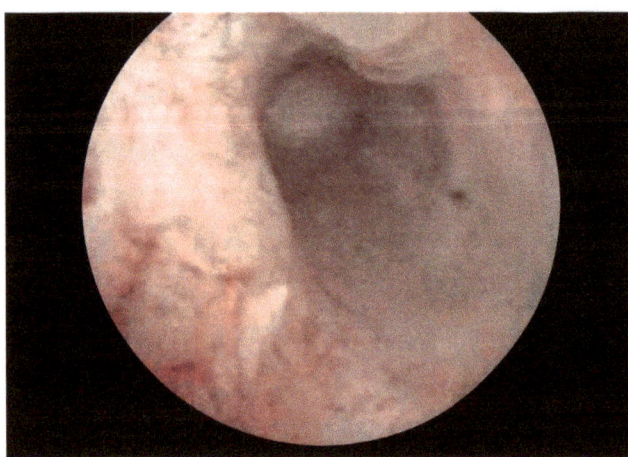

Fig. 10: Hysteroscopic view of Robert's uterus.

AUTHOR'S EXPERIENCE

Study at Ramakrishna Medical Centre LLP, Trichy (2011–2018; Flowchart 1)

- Incidence of Müllerian anomalies is (120/1,182 laparoscopic surgeries) 9.3%.
- Mayer-Rokitansky-Küster-Hauser syndrome five cases (no endometriosis).
- Unicornuate uterus nine cases (no endometriosis).
- Bicornuate and didelphys uterus 12 cases (eight had endometriosis)—66%.
- Septate uterus 96 cases (16 had endometriosis) 17%.
- 24/120—20% had endometriosis among Müllerian anomalies.

Müllerian Anomalies and Endometriosis

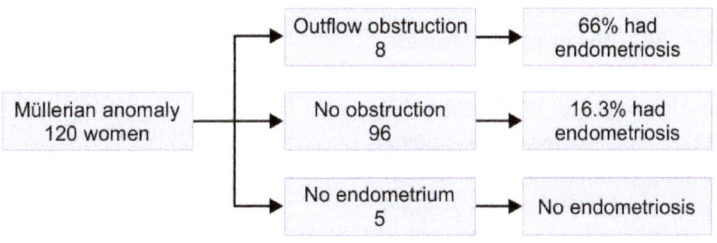

Flowchart 1: Ramakrishna experience.

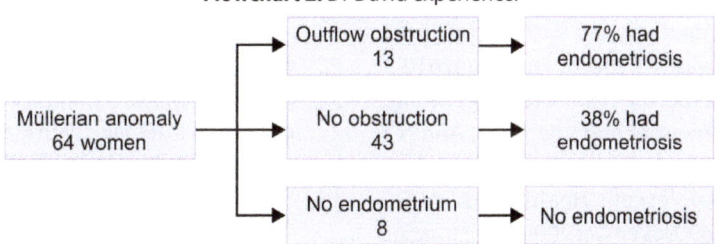

Flowchart 2: Dr David experience.

There was a study by Dr David and Dr Henderson in the literature regarding endometriosis and Müllerian anomalies published in the year 1987 (Flowchart 2).
- Twenty-six out of 64 cases had endometriosis giving an incidence of 40.6%.

CONCLUSION

Müllerian anomalies are significantly associated with endometriosis. Early diagnosis and treatment improves menstrual and reproductive outcome. Both medical and surgical therapies play a significant role in treatment. Endometriosis usually does not recur after treatment of the obstruction. Early detection, definite intervention, and long-term follow-up help to prevent the recurrence of endometriosis and promote fertility.

REFERENCES

1. Fukunaga T, Fujii S, Inoue C, et al. The spectrum of imaging appearances of Müllerian duct anomalies: focus on MR imaging. Jpn J Radiol. 2017;35(12):697-706.
2. Fedele L, Bianchi S, Di Nola G, et al. Endometriosis and nonobstructive Müllerian anomalies. Obstet Gynecol. 1992;79(4):515-7.
3. Rackow BW, Arici A. Reproductive performance of women with Müllerian anomalies. Curr Opin Obstet Gynecol. 2007;19(3):229-37.
4. Uğur M, Turan C, Mungan T, et al. Endometriosis in association with Müllerian anomalies. Gynecol Obstet Invest. 1995;40(4):261-4.
5. Du H, Taylor HS. The role of Hox genes in female reproductive tract development, adult function, and fertility. Cold Spring Harb Perspect Med. 2016;6(1):a023002.
6. Cramer DW, Hornstein MD, Ng WG, et al. Endometriosis associated with the N314D mutation of galactose-1-phosphate uridyltransferase (GALT). Mol Hum Reprod. 1996; 2(3):149-52.
7. Bhagavath B, Ellie G, Griffiths KM, et al. Uterine malformations: An update of diagnosis, management, and outcomes. Obstet Gynecol Surv. 2017;72(6):377-92.
8. Dreisler E, Stampe Sørensen S. Müllerian duct anomalies diagnosed by saline contrast sonohysterography: prevalence in a general population. Fertil Steril. 2014; 102(2):525-9.
9. Appelman Z, Hazan Y, Hagay Z. High prevalence of Müllerian anomalies diagnosed by ultrasound in women with polycystic ovaries. J Reprod Med. 2003;48(5):362-4.
10. Li S, Qayyum A, Coakley FV, et al. Association of renal agenesis and Müllerian duct anomalies. J Comput Assist Tomogr. 2000;24(6):829-34.
11. Kapczuk K, Friebe Z, Iwaniec K, et al. Obstructive Müllerian Anomalies in Menstruating Adolescent Girls: A Report of 22 Cases. J Pediatr Adolesc Gynecol. 2018;31(3):252-7.
12. Rock JA. Anomalous development of the vagina. Semin Reprod Endocrinol. 1986;4:13.
13. Laufer MR. Structural abnormalities of the female reproductive tract. Emans, Laufer, Goldstein's Pediatric and Adolescent Gynecology, 6th edition. Philadelphia: Lippincott Williams and Wilkins; 2012. p. 334.

14. Heinonen PK. Unicornuate uterus and rudimentary horn. Fertil Steril. 1997;68(2):224-30.
15. Fujimoto VY, Klein NA, Miller PB. Late-onset hematometra and hematosalpinx in a woman with a noncommunicating uterine horn. A case report. J Reprod Med. 1998;43(5):465-7.
16. Kamio M, Nagata T, Yamasaki H, Yoshinaga M, et al. Inguinal hernia containing functioning, rudimentary uterine horn and endometriosis. Obstet Gynecol. 2009;113(2 Pt 2):563-6.
17. Nawroth F, Rahimi G, Nawroth C, et al. Is there an association between septate uterus and endometriosis? Hum Reprod. 2006;21(2):542-4.
18. LaMonica R, Pinto J, Luciano D. Incidence of septate uterus in reproductive-aged women with and without endometriosis. J Minim Invasive Gynecol. 2016;23(4):610-3.
19. Leyendecker G, Kunz G, Herbertz M, et al. Uterine peristaltic activity and the development of endometriosis. Ann N Y Acad Sci. 2004;1034,338-55.
20. ACOG Committee on Adolescent Health Care. ACOG Committee Opinion No. 349, November 2006: Menstruation in girls and adolescents: using the menstrual cycle as a vital sign. Obstet Gynecol. 2006;108(5):1323-8.
21. Cox D, Ching BH. Herlyn-Werner-Wunderlich syndrome: a rare presentation with pyocolpos. J Radiol Case Rep. 2012; 6(3):9-15.
22. Dietrich JE, Millar DM, Quint EH. Obstructive reproductive tract anomalies. J Pediatr Adolesc Gynecol. 2014;27(6): 396-402.
23. Santos XM, Krishnamurthy R, Bercaw-Pratt JL, et al. The utility of ultrasound and magnetic resonance imaging versus surgery for the characterization of Müllerian anomalies in the pediatric and adolescent population. J Pediatr Adolesc Gynecol. 2012;25(3):181-4.
24. Krüger K, Behrendt Niedobitek-Kreuter G, Koltermann K, et al. Location-dependent value of pelvic MRI in the preoperative diagnosis of endometriosis. Eur J Obstet Gynecol Reprod Biol. 2013;169(1):93-8.
25. Elliott JE, Abduljabar H, Morris M. Presurgical management of dysmenorrhea and endometriosis in a patient with Mayer-Rokitansky-Kuster-Hauser syndrome. Fertil Steril. 2011;96(2):e86-9.
26. Bailez MM. Laparoscopy in uterovaginal anomalies. Semin Pediatr Surg. 2007;16(4):278-87.
27. Silveira SA, Laufer MR. Persistence of endometriosis after correction of an obstructed reproductive tract anomaly. J Pediatr Adolesc Gynecol. 2013;26(4):e93-4.
28. Marsh CA, Will MA, Smorgick N, et al. Uterine remnants and pelvic pain in females with Mayer-Rokitansky-Küster-Hauser syndrome. J Pediatr Adolesc Gynecol. 2013;26(3):199-202.
29. Wang Y, Lu J, Zhu L, et al. Evaluation of Mayer-Rokitansky-Küster-Hauser syndrome with magnetic resonance imaging: Three patterns of uterine remnants and related anatomical features and clinical settings. Eur Radiol. 2017;27(12):5215-24.
30. Aveiro AC, Miranda V, Cabral AJ, et al. Herlyn-Werner-Wunderlich syndrome: a rare cause of pelvic pain in adolescent girls. BMJ Case Rep. 2011.
31. Khaladkar SM, Kamal V, Kamal A, et al. The Herlyn-Werner-Wunderlich Syndrome—A case report with radiological review. Pol J Radiol. 2016;81:395-400.
32. Sardeshpande N, Chipalkatti P, Doctor J. Robert's uterus: a rare congenital anomaly. Int J Reprod Contracept Obstet Gynecol. 2017;6(12):5657-9.

CHAPTER 7

Stimulation in Endometriosis and Adenomyosis: Is it Different?

Abha Majumdar, Neeti Tiwari

INTRODUCTION

Endometriosis is a disease of unknown origin, which is inflammatory in nature and manifests as pelvic pain and/or infertility. The incidence of endometriosis in women of reproductive age group in general population is approximately 10% whereas in infertile women the incidence increases to about 40–50%.[1] Adenomyosis is often associated with endometriosis, and in these cases there is further decline in fertility by even lower endometrial receptivity by interference to endometrial blood flow by the adenomyotic lesions. Endometriosis is classically diagnosed on laparoscopy and histopathology of biopsied specimens. Since laparoscopy may not be warranted in all cases of infertility, transvaginal ultrasound (TVS) and magnetic resonance imaging (MRI) have emerged as important diagnostic tools and are highly sensitive and specific for endometriomas and deep infiltrating lesions. However, superficial lesions evade diagnosis by these imaging modalities and can only be diagnosed by direct visualization on laparoscopy.[2] Assisted reproductive technology (ART) is now the preferred and ultimate treatment of endometriosis related infertility. Surgery finds a role in endometriosis in the younger women with brief period of infertility, good ovarian reserve, spontaneous ovulation, and normal semen parameters as it enhances the chances of natural conception if tubes are patent and tubo-ovarian relationship has been restored. After laparoscopy the couple is advised to try natural conception for 6–12 months and if they fail to conceive during this period, one may consider ART. In older couples with long-standing infertility, low ovarian reserve, and advanced disease, ART should be offered directly, as laparoscopic cystectomy offers no benefit in this group and may rather reduce their chances of conception by further reducing their ovarian reserve.[3] The exception to this rule is presence of large endometrioma which may interfere with follicular aspiration or presence of connecting hydrosalpinx which could reduce the implantation potential of the embryo. Numerous studies in literature have reported poorer outcomes in in vitro fertilization (IVF) in women with endometriosis as compared to tubal factor infertility. We need to understand the challenges with endometriosis and adenomyosis so that the stimulation protocols can be tailored to get best possible results from ART in this subset of patients.

CHALLENGES IN ENDOMETRIOSIS

In a retrospective cohort study 431 cycles in women with endometriosis were compared with 596 with tubal factor infertility. Patients with endometriosis required higher doses and longer duration of gonadotropins, still the number of oocytes and good quality embryos was lower than tubal factor infertility. Implantation rates were also found to be lower in endometriosis. However, clinical pregnancy rates, miscarriage rates, and live birth rates were not significantly lower in endometriosis.[4] Another retrospective cohort study which compared IVF outcomes in women with endometriosis (n = 531) to those with unexplained infertility (n = 737) found lower live birth rate in endometriosis group after single embryo transfer [OR 0.76 (95% CI, 0.59–0.98) P = 0.035].[5] A "dose-response relationship" was seen as the effect of endometriosis on reproductive outcomes was found to be greater with increasing disease severity. Nevertheless, a recent large retrospective cohort study where IVF outcomes of 3,583 women with endometriosis were compared to 18,833 controls, no difference was found in terms of clinical pregnancy rates, miscarriage rates, and pregnancy rates within the two groups. Although the average number of oocytes retrieved were less in endometriosis group the percentage of fertilized oocytes were not different.[6]

Different studies have shown varied results regarding the effect of endometriosis on ART outcomes. Since endometriosis is a chronic inflammatory disorder which involves both ovaries and uterus it poses unique challenges as compared to other causes of infertility.

- *Low ovarian reserve*: Women with endometriosis are likely to have lower ovarian reserve as compared to their age-matched controls. The pathology of endometriosis per se reduces the ovarian reserve and then the surgical treatment, i.e. ovarian cystectomy and adhesiolysis takes further toll on normal ovarian tissues. The exceptions are only women where both endometriosis and polycystic ovarian syndrome coexist. During controlled ovarian stimulation in cases of endometriosis usually higher doses and longer duration of gonadotropins are required.
- *Poor oocyte quality*: Endometriosis has been associated with poor oocyte quality subsequently leading to poor embryogenesis. In a prospective controlled study mature metaphase II (MII) mouse oocytes were divided in two groups, in the test group the oocytes were cultured in peritoneal fluid of women with endometriosis and in the control group they were cultured in the peritoneal fluid of women undergoing tubal ligation. In the test group significantly more microtubule aberrations and chromosomal changes in the mouse oocytes were seen as compared to control group.[7] In a case control study 431 IVF cycles in women with endometriosis were compared with 2,510 cycles in other factors. The oocyte yield and number of embryos obtained were less in endometriosis group but pregnancy rate and miscarriage rate did not significantly differ. The incidence of extracytoplasmic oocyte defects were also found to be higher in endometriosis group.[8] In a donor recipient model it was shown that when donor oocytes were taken for women with low ovarian reserve with endometriosis no difference was found in implantation and pregnancy rates in recipient women with endometriosis as compared to others if donors were free of endometriosis. On the other hand, when oocytes were retrieved from donors with endometriosis there was significant reduction in implantation rate. The authors suggested that in endometriosis there could be alterations in oocyte quality which leads to embryos with low implantation potential.[9]
- *Impaired implantation*: Reduced endometrial receptivity has been considered as one of the factors causing infertility in endometriosis though mechanism is not clear. Integrin $\alpha5\beta3$, a cell adhesion molecule which has a prime role in implantation, was shown to have reduced expression in endometrium of some women with endometriosis.[10] Recently, decreased levels of enzymes involved in synthesis of endometrial ligand for L-selectin, a protein that coats the trophoblast on the surface of blastocyst, have been observed in endometriotic women.[11] But later many studies based on oocyte donation program found that implantation rates and pregnancy rates are similar in recipients with or without endometriosis irrespective of the severity of disease. Endometrial receptivity assay (ERA) of infertile women with and without endometriosis also showed similar gene signaling irrespective of the stage of disease.[12] Hence, it can be concluded that poor IVF outcomes in endometriosis are mainly due to poor oocyte quality and impaired embryogenesis, endometrial factor even if present can be overcome with good quality embryos.

CONSIDERATIONS WHEN PLANNING A PROTOCOL FOR IVF IN ENDOMETRIOSIS

The aim of an ideal protocol in endometriosis is to get good number of high-quality oocytes with the best possible endometrium for transfer. Following considerations should be kept in mind while planning IVF in women with endometriosis:
- Age of the women and duration of infertility
- Ovarian reserve [serum anti-Müllerian hormone (AMH) and antral follicle count on TVS]
- Stage of endometriosis: Stage 1 and 2 are managed as unexplained while stage 3 and 4 as pelvic-tubal factor
- Presence of other confounding factors responsible for infertility.

Ultra-long Protocol: The Ideal Protocol for Endometriosis

Suppression of endometriosis by prolonged administration of gonadotropin releasing hormone (GnRH) agonist may improve oocyte quality, embryo quality and thus, indirectly the implantation rates. A systematic review (2006) of three randomized controlled trials (RCTs) including 165 women concluded that administration of GnRH agonists for a period of 3-6 months prior to IVF or intracytoplasmic sperm injection (ICSI) cycle increases the odds of clinical pregnancy fourfold and live birth rate ninefold.[13] The reason behind better pregnancy rates with prolonged pituitary suppression in endometriosis is not yet clear. Different novel mechanisms have been proposed by which GnRH agonists work on endometriosis:

- Suppression of ovulation by GnRH agonists reduces exposure of endometriotic implants to growth factor *midkine* present in follicular fluid which is involved in proliferation of endometriotic implants.
- There is a direct inhibition of proliferation of endometriotic implants by regulation of angiogenic and apoptotic factors.
- Inhibition of menstruation reduces exposure to thrombin and its protease-activated receptor; factor which leads to cell inflammation.
- Inhibition of uterine contractions also blocks mechanical stress.

Prolonged downregulation is associated with certain pitfalls. It is a time-consuming protocol and sometimes it profoundly dampens the ovarian response to stimulation leading to longer and greater requirement of gonadotropins.[14] Cycle cancellations are higher due to poor response after prolonged suppression in women with already compromised ovarian reserve in endometriosis. Long-term use of GnRH agonists is also associated with side effects such as vasomotor instability and bone loss. Hence, conventional protocols like GnRH agonist long protocol and antagonist are being widely used for women with endometriosis also.

Antagonist versus Long Protocol in Endometriosis

Gonadotropin-releasing hormone agonist long protocol is a time-tested protocol but is associated with longer duration of injections, higher dose of gonadotropins and increased risk of ovarian hyperstimulation syndrome (OHSS). Antagonist protocol on the other hand is more patient friendly and has reduced risk of OHSS may also offer an advantage in women with limited ovarian reserve because of its mechanism of action. In a prospective randomized trial on 246 patients with mild-moderate endometriosis undergoing IVF-ICSI, no difference was found in implantation rates and clinical pregnancy rates when GnRH antagonist or GnRH agonist long protocol was used. The number of MII oocytes and available embryos though were higher in long protocol group leading to higher cumulative pregnancy rates after frozen transfer in this group.[15] However, with the learning curve of using antagonist protocols, recent trials comparing both protocols showed similar IVF outcomes in terms of positive pregnancy rates (25% vs. 21.4% p 0.269) and ongoing pregnancy rates (20.5% vs. 19.1% p 0.302) in patients with severe endometriosis and past history of laparoscopy.[16]

Pretreatment with Standard Protocols

- *Pretreatment with oral contraceptive pills*: Oral contraceptive pills (OCPs) have been widely used as pretreatment before antagonist cycle for synchronization of follicular cohort but its effect on pregnancy rates has been controversial. Geisinger et al. (2008) after a systematic review and meta-analysis concluded that a significant decrease in ongoing pregnancy rates was seen when pretreatment with oral contraceptives was given in antagonist cycles.[14] In endometriosis due to the basic pathology pretreatment with OCPs may prove beneficial. In a pilot trial (2010) the results indicated that 6-8 weeks of continuous OCPs intake prior to IVF in patients of endometriosis not only improves outcome but possibly appeared equally effective as GnRH agonist treatment. The authors presumed that the beneficial effect of OCPs could be due to improved endometrial receptivity or effect on oocyte quality.[17] A noninferiority RCT is underway to compare continuous OCPs versus prolonged down regulation prior to IVF or ICSI in moderate to severe endometriosis.
- *Pretreatment with letrozole*: Aromatase inhibitors reduce peripheral estrogen levels by preventing aromatization of androgenic precursors, a mechanism different from GnRH agonists. Letrozole and GnRH agonists have been used together to alleviate endometriosis associated pain. A retrospective cohort study on 126 women with endometriomas who had one failed IVF was conducted to see if this combination gives them better outcome in ART. The test group received pretreatment with two doses of leuprolide acetate depot 3.75 mg 1 month apart with 60 days tab letrozole 5 mg while control group only received leuprolide depot. When IVF was done the dose of gonadotropins used was significantly less and number of mature oocytes were more in the letrozole group. The clinical pregnancy rate and live birth rate were also significantly higher in the test group.[18]

OVARIAN STIMULATION AND ENDOMETRIOSIS RECURRENCE

The peripheral estrogen levels rise considerably in ART cycles and often reach a level which is ten times higher than natural cycle. Since endometriosis is considered to be an estrogen dependent condition, there is a pertinent question in the minds of both clinicians and patients regarding progression and recurrence of endometriosis after ovarian stimulation. A recently published systematic review of 16 studies addressed this issue and came out with following conclusions:[19]

- Endometriosis related pain is not worsened by IVF
- IVF does not increase the risk of recurrence of endometriosis
- A mild increase, if at all may occur in the size of endometriomas after IVF (low quality evidence)
- Intrauterine insemination (IUI) may increase risk of recurrence (low quality evidence)
- Deep endometriosis may get worsened by IVF (very low-quality evidence).

SEGMENTED APPROACH IN IVF FOR PATIENTS WITH ENDOMETRIOSIS

In order to limit the risk of disease flaring and optimize the results, segmentation of IVF with antagonist protocol, agonist trigger and elective freezing of embryos has been proposed by some authors.[20] Since ultra-long protocol sometimes leads to profound suppression of ovarian response in endometriosis, retrieving oocytes in an antagonist cycle, freezing all embryos and then transferring after prolonged pituitary down regulation has shown excellent outcomes.[21]

CONCLUSION

Adequate and safe ovarian stimulation is the basis of a successful ART program. Therefore, optimizing stimulation in women going in for IVF with any indication, more so in an ovarian inflammatory condition such as endometriosis, may benefit the eventual ART outcome. Hence, individualization of controlled ovarian stimulation protocols in women with endometriosis especially in advanced stages of the disease may give the best chances of pregnancy and live birth.

REFERENCES

1. Eisenberg VH, Weil C, Chodick G, et al. Epidemiology of endometriosis: a large population based study from a healthcare provider with 2 million members. BJOG. 2018;125(1):55-62.
2. Nisenblat V, Bossuyt M, Farquhar C, et al. Imaging modalities for the non-invasive diagnosis of endometriosis. Cochrane Database Sys Rev. 2016;2:CD009591.
3. Hamdan M, Dunselman G, Li TC, et al. The impact of endometrioma on IVF/ICSI outcome: a systematic review and meta-analysis. Hum Reprod Update. 2015;20:633-43.
4. Dong X, Liao X, Wang R, et al. The impact of endometriosis on IVF/ICSI outcomes. Int J Clin Exp Pathol. 2013;6(9):1911-8.
5. Muteshi CM, Ohuma EO, Child T, et al. The effect of endometriosis on live birth rate and other reproductive outcomes in ART cycles: a cohort study. Hum Reprod Open. 2018;2018(4):16.
6. González Comadran M, Schwarze JE, Zegers-Hochschild F, et al. The impact of endometriosis on outcome of Assisted Reproductive Technology. Reprod Biol Endocrinol. 2017;15(1):8.
7. Monsur G, Sharma R, Lofty G, et al. Endometriosis induced changes in mouse oocyte cytoskeleton. Fertil Steril. 2007;82(Suppl 1):S207.
8. Borges E, Braga DP, Setti AS, et al. The influence of endometriosis on oocyte quality and embryo developmental competence. Fertil Steril. 2015;104(3):e201-e202.
9. Simón C, Gutiérrez A, Vidal A, et al. Outcome of patients with endometriosis in assisted reproduction: results from in-vitro fertilization and oocyte donation. Hum Reprod. 1994;9(4):725-9.
10. Lessey BA, Castelbaum AJ, Sawin SW, et al. Aberrant integrin expression in the endometrium of women with endometriosis. J Clin Endocrinol Metab. 1994;79(2):643-9.
11. Burney RO, Talbi S, Hamilton AE, et al. Gene expression analysis of endometrium reveals progesterone resistance and candidate susceptibility genes in women with endometriosis. Endocrinology. 2007;48(8):3814-26.
12. Velanciano JM, Alonso MR, Gómez E, et al. Endometrial receptivity in eutopic endometrium in patients with endometriosis: it is not affected, and let me show you why. Fertil Steril. 2017;108(1):28-31.
13. Sallam HN, Gracia-Velasco JA, Dias S, et al. Long-term pituitary down-regulation before in in vitro fertilization (IVF) for women with endometriosis. Cochrane Database Syst Rev. 2006;25(1):CD004635.
14. Griesinger G, Venetis CA, Marx T, et al. Oral contraceptive pill pretreatment in ovarian stimulation with GnRH antagonists for IVF: a systematic review and meta-analysis. Fertil Steril. 2008;90(4):1055-63.

15. Pabuccu R, Onalan G, Kaya C. GnRH agonist and antagonist protocols for mild-moderate endometriosis and endometrioma in in-vitro fertilization/intracytoplasmic sperm injection cycles. Fertil Steril. 2007;88(4):832-9.
16. Bastu E, Yasa C, Dural O, et al. Comparison of ovulation induction protocols after endometrioma resection. JSLS. 2014;18(3):e2014.00128.
17. de Ziegler D, Gayet V, Aubriot FX, et al. Use of oral contraceptive pills in women with endometriosis before assisted reproductive treatment improves outcomes. Fertil Steril. 2010;94(7):2796-9.
18. Cantor A, Tannus S, San WY, et al. A comparison of two months pretreatment with GnRH agonists with or without an aromatase inhibitor in women with ultrasound-diagnosed ovarian endometriomas undergoing IVF. Reprod Biomed Online. 2019;38(4):520-7.
19. Somigliana E, Viganò P, Benaglia L, et al. Ovarian stimulation and endometriosis progression or recurrence: a systematic review. Reprod Biomed Online. 2019;38(2):185-94.
20. de Ziegler D, Pirtea P, Carbonnel M, et al. Assisted reproduction in endometriosis. Best Practice and Research Clinical Endocrinology and metabolism. 2019;33(1):47-59.
21. Surrey ES, Jaffe MK, Kondapalli LV, et al. GnRH agonist administration prior to embryo transfer in freeze-all cycles with endometriosis or aberrant integrin expression. Reprod Biomed Online. 2017;35(2):145-51.

CHAPTER 8

Tips of Surgery in Endometriosis

Nutan Jain

INTRODUCTION

Endometriosis is an enigmatic disease. In the recent times, lot of attention has been given to elucidating the exact nature, etiopathology, and disease symptomatology in relation to chronic pelvic pain. Deep infiltrating endometriosis has been directly related to pelvic pain, dysmenorrhea, and dyspareunia. Laparoscopy has emerged as a major player in the diagnosis and especially for surgical management of deep infiltrating endometriosis (Fig. 1).

Conquer endometriosis means to conquer pain and infertility.

Medical therapy is found to be ineffective and temporary with recurrence rate as high as 76%[1] whereas surgical treatment is highly effective in relieving pelvic pain and dyspareunia. The old concept of hysterectomy and bilateral salpingo-oophorectomy in relieving pain is ineffective in the face of deep infiltrating endometriosis of rectovaginal space and uterosacral ligaments.

For all endometriotic surgeries, we use 5 mm trocar via Jain point and optimize 10 mm telescope according to surgery. The Jain point is located in the left paraumbilical region at the level of umbilicus, on a straight line drawn vertically upward from a point 2.5 cm medial to anterior superior iliac spine (ASIS).[2]

After visualizing lesion of ovary/rectovaginal septum, etc. we inject pitressin in dilution of 20 units in 300 mL normal saline (NS). It is very useful for decreasing intraoperative blood loss as well as making dissection planes easier. All endometriosis procedures include peritoneal washing for cytology, inspection of pelvis and peritoneal organs, and adhesiolysis.

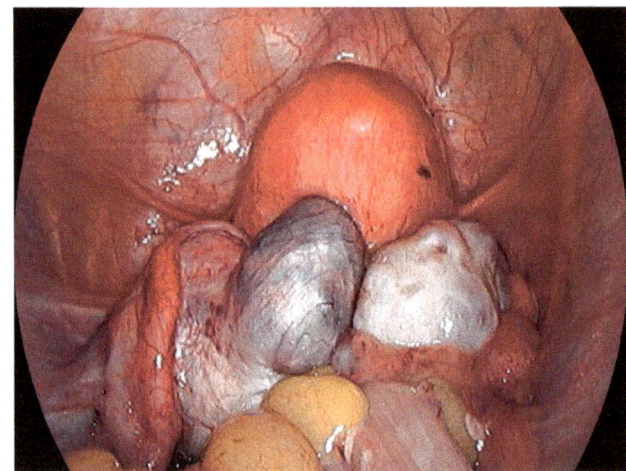

Fig. 1: Deep infiltrating endometriosis with bilateral kissing ovaries.

MAIN SITES FOR ENDOMETRIOSIS

The main sites for endometriosis are:
- Peritoneal endometriosis
- Endometrioma of ovary
- Rectovaginal endometriosis
- Endometriosis of urinary bladder/ureter
- Retrocervical and bowel endometriosis.

Peritoneal Endometriosis

It is of three types:
- *Type I lesions* are usually large subtle conical lesions surrounded by white sclerotic tissue.
- *Type II lesions* are small in size and are formed by retraction of the bowel. Sometimes, these lesions are

only marked by induration. On excision of such a lesion, a nodule can also be revealed.³
- *Type III disease* or deep infiltrating endometriosis (DIE) is the most severe form of peritoneal disease which is marked by painful nodularities at the time of rectovaginal examination and is due to involvement of the rectovaginal septum.² It usually presents as chronic pelvic pain, severe dysmenorrhea, and/or deep dyspareunia. The diagnosis of DIE can be easily made through clinical examination; however it may be sometimes missed, when it particularly involves smaller areas which can only be diagnosed at laparoscopy as typical lesions or as dark blue cysts at the vaginal fornix. Diagnosis in such cases may be enhanced if clinical examination is performed during menstruation which can be further supported by transrectal or vaginal ultrasound examination or MR imaging. CA-125 levels performed during menstruation can also help in diagnosing deep infiltrating disease.⁴ Levels above 35 U/mL are associated with endometriosis with a low sensitivity of 36% and a fairly high specificity of 87%.⁵

Treatment of deep infiltrating disease is most commonly surgical resection of the disease by following the tissue planes between normal tissue and the nodule. Lesions 5–6 mm in size are generally flat, whereas deep lesions are usually elongated. Complete excision may be successfully performed laparoscopically in majority of the cases, however vaginal excision may also be needed in few. Particular concern of not damaging the ureter should always be kept in mind while performing the surgery in cases of DIE. Thus, we always perform retroperitoneal dissection to delineate the full pelvic course of the ureters. However, at times, it could be hard time dissecting out the right planes. In such cases, possibility of encountering an acute or remote ureteric injury may be high, thus prophylactic ureteric stenting is highly recommended. The availability of trans-illuminating ureteric stents and indocyanine green dye has made it an easy job to identify and save the ureters from injury during difficult dissections. Whether the dissection is accomplished with a CO_2 laser harmonics or sharp scissors, is a matter of personal preference. Many surgeons choose not to use electrosurgery because of the associated widespread thermal damage and difficulty in recognizing tissue planes (Figs. 2 to 5).

Ablation of endometriotic implants: Vaporization or fulguration of all endometriotic implants on back surface of uterus, cervix, and uterosacral ligaments is carried out after

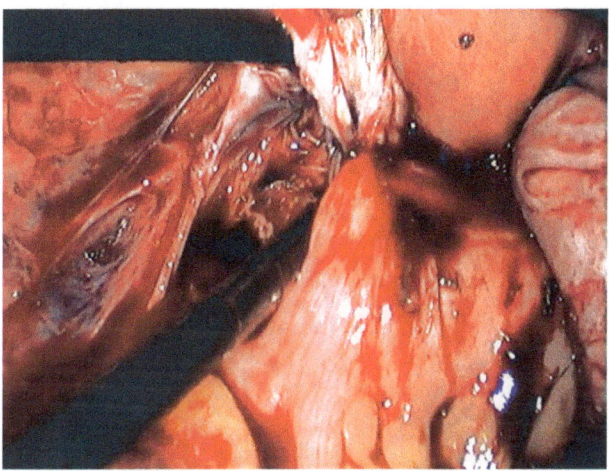
Fig. 2: Excision of rectovaginal nodule.

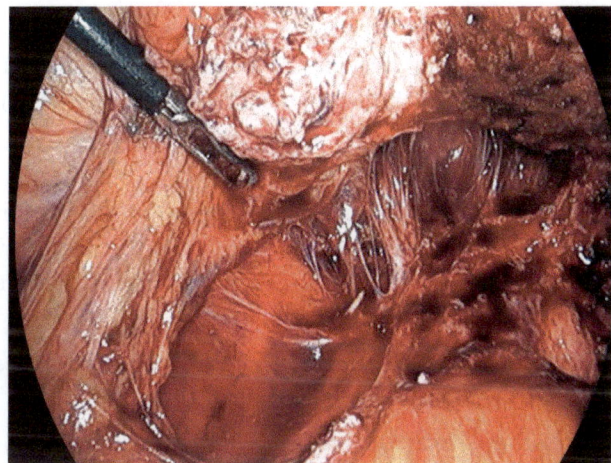
Fig. 3: Rectal mobilization and ureteric dissection in deep infiltrating endometriosis.

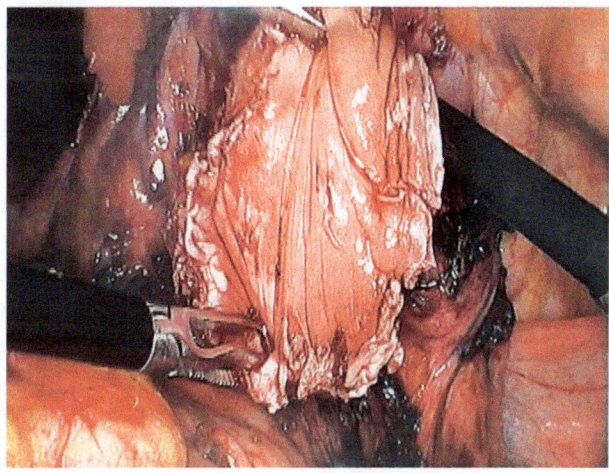
Fig. 4: Excised rectovaginal nodule.

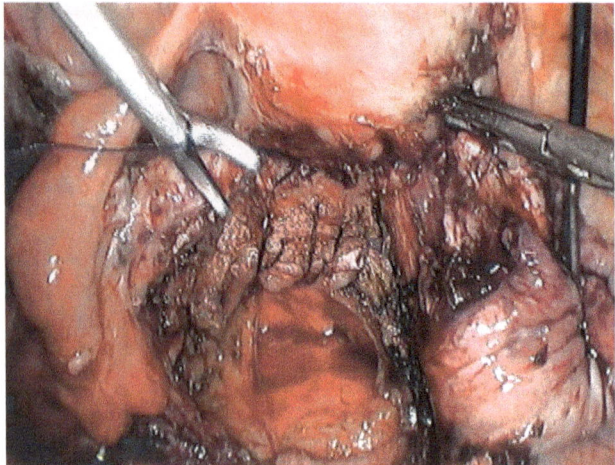

Fig. 5: Final appearance of pelvis after suturing of excised nodule.

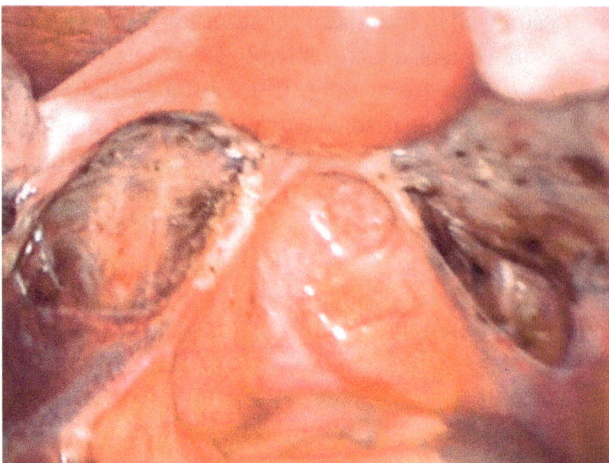

Fig. 6: Fulguration of peritoneal endometriosis.

rectal mobilization, lateral clearing and excising nodule using microbipolar forceps. Thorough suction irrigation lavage is done and complete hemostasis is achieved (Fig. 6).

Endometrioma

With sonographic evaluation, taking in consideration the revised AFS classification, 1985, it can be classified according to the extension of disease from minimal to severe endometriosis (stage I to IV) as follows:

Minimal endometriosis (stage I): There are minimal chances of growth of endometrial tissue outside the uterus.

Mild endometriosis (stage II): Mono- or bilateral endometriomas with diameter <3 cm; ovaries in normal site, mobile, and not adherent to the uterus and surrounding tissues.

Moderate endometriosis (stage III): Mono- or bilateral endometriomas with diameter >3 cm; at least one ovary in normal site, mobile, and not adherent to the uterus and surrounding tissues or one ovary only adherent to the uterus or broad ligament.

Severe endometriosis (stage IV): Mono- or bilateral endometriomas with diameter >3 cm; ovaries in abnormal site (prolapsed in the pouch of Douglas or dislocated posteriorly, anteriorly or superiorly to the uterus) and adherent to the uterus and surrounding tissues; presence of pelvic adhesions or endometriotic nodules.

For endometrioma of ovary, laser vaporization of cyst or cyst enucleation can be done.

Pitressin is injected between the cyst wall and ovarian capsule which helps in delineating the plane. Then with the

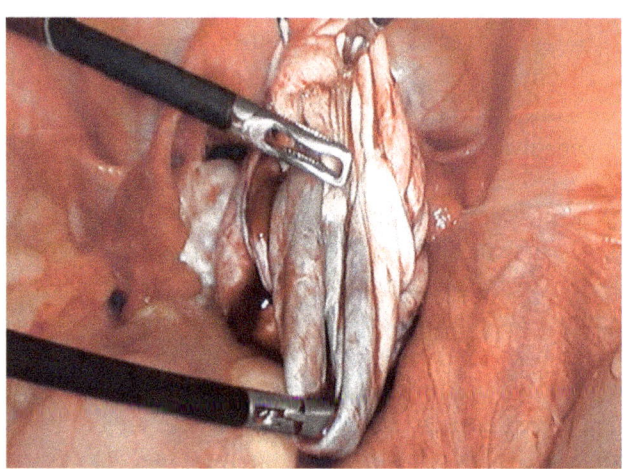

Fig. 7: Cyst enucleation of endometrioma of ovary.

help of two graspers, one holds the ovary and another strips off the cyst lining (Fig. 7).

Surgical Technique

The technique for endometriotic cystectomy followed at our hospital is described in Flowchart 1.

Endometriosis of Rectovaginal Septum

It involves management of adhesions and pain.

Adhesiolysis

- Complete dissection of anterior rectum with blunt hook/scissors until the loose fibro-fatty tissues is reached.
- Open peritoneum covering cul-de-sac between adenomyotic lesion and rectum.
- Excise deep endometriosis.

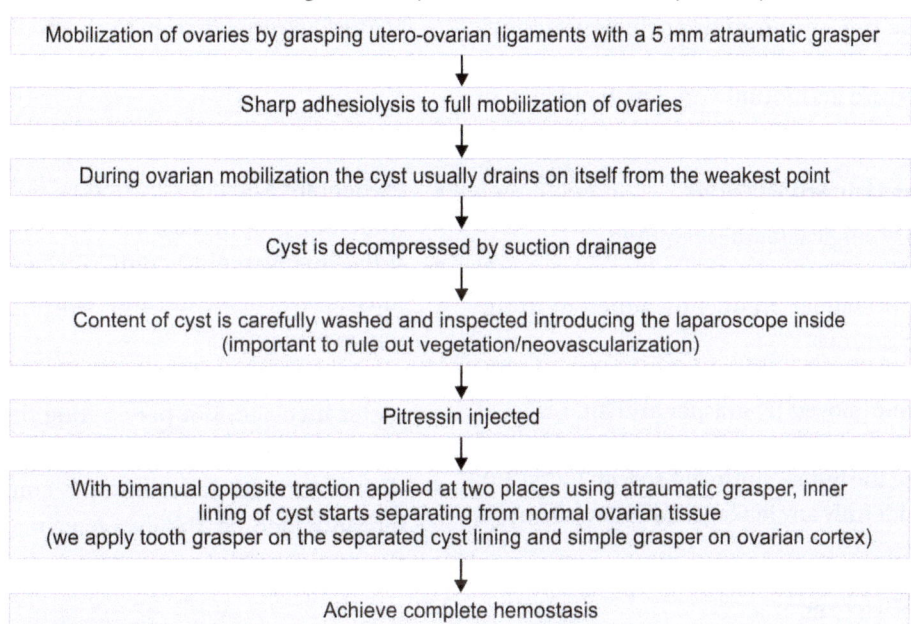

Flowchart 1: Surgical technique used for endometriotic cystectomy.

```
Mobilization of ovaries by grasping utero-ovarian ligaments with a 5 mm atraumatic grasper
                                    ↓
            Sharp adhesiolysis to full mobilization of ovaries
                                    ↓
    During ovarian mobilization the cyst usually drains on itself from the weakest point
                                    ↓
                   Cyst is decompressed by suction drainage
                                    ↓
  Content of cyst is carefully washed and inspected introducing the laparoscope inside
            (important to rule out vegetation/neovascularization)
                                    ↓
                            Pitressin injected
                                    ↓
  With bimanual opposite traction applied at two places using atraumatic grasper, inner
              lining of cyst starts separating from normal ovarian tissue
   (we apply tooth grasper on the separated cyst lining and simple grasper on ovarian cortex)
                                    ↓
                        Achieve complete hemostasis
```

Pain

Clearing between uterosacral ligaments and rectum as it carries afferent nerves for pain. We identify and lateralize the inferior hypogastric plexus. We also trace and lateralize pelvic ureter. Excise uterosacral ligaments. Vagina if involved: excise the adenomyotic nodule with 0.5 cm disease free margin. En-bloc excision by monopolar cautery/harmonic is done and sutured with 1-0 vicryl (Figs. 8 and 9).

Rectal excision (Partial/full thickness): It is not practiced commonly as there is difficulty in obtaining consent and explanation of need of colostomy in eventuality of a mishap in radical rectal excision; we prefer *"radical reproductive surgeries"* and mobilize rectum from posterior surface of uterus, do the lateral clearing and excision of adenomyotic nodules, referring from unnecessary radial rectal resection.

Adhesion Prevention

After such extensive dissection, concern for postoperative adhesion formation is real. Use of Interceed® is propagated by many. Use of fluid barriers is also widespread, like 4% icodextrin. In our setup we prefer to use fluid adhesion barriers and 4% icodextrin is our choice. At times we use only Ringer's lactate and as per Reich et al. practice instill 3 L at end of such extensive procedure.[6] Patients complain of some bloating for 24 hours after hydrofloatation but

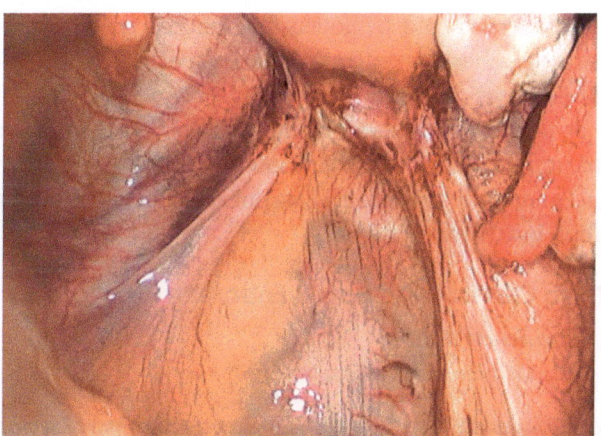

Fig. 8: Endometriosis of rectovaginal septum.

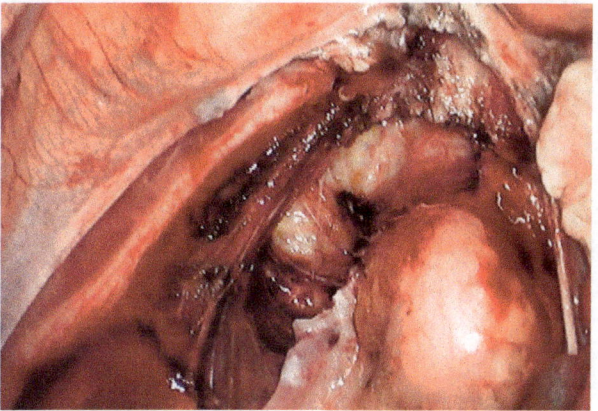

Fig. 9: Nerve dissection for nerve sparing surgery.

otherwise they tolerate it well. The principle of hydrofloatation works by prevention of opposing surfaces to adhere to each other. On at least three patients we did a second-look procedure and found very low incidence of re-adhesion formation.

Endometriosis of Urinary Bladder

- Multidisciplinary surgical team is required.
- *Bladder*: Bladder lesions are usually located in roof/posterior wall of bladder, frequently adherent to the uterine corpus/isthmus.

Preliminary cystoscopy is done to identify endometriotic lesions. Lesions are removed by grasper and are resected either mechanically with scissors or monopolar pure cut mode. After excising the lesion, suture these with Vicryl 3-0. Distend it again to identify any leakage. Catheter is kept for 7–14 days (Fig. 10).

Endometriosis of Ureter

First identify for extrinsic compression distortion of anatomy/intrinsic disease. Ureter is exposed in its entire length. Adhesiolysis is done without using electrical energy. Excise extrinsic adhesions/intrinsic lesion. For extensive lesion—adhesiolysis and sharp scissor dissection is done. For deep intrinsic lesion—segmental excision and end-to-end anastomosis with 5-0 monofilament is done.

For ureteric stricture at lower one-third, ureteric implantation into bladder is done.

Retro Cervical and Bowel Endometriosis

- *Incidence*: 3–37%[7]
- *Rectosigmoid involvement*: 90%[8]

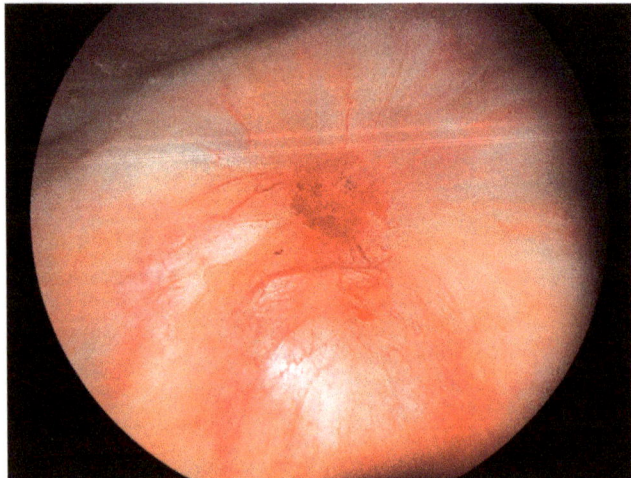

Fig. 10: Bladder endometriosis.

- *Required investigation*: TVS/MRI
- Multidisciplinary approach involving a colorectal surgeon is required.

Steps

- Preoperative bowel preparation.
- Antibiotic prophylaxis.
- If the involvement is only serosa or only superficial muscle layer of rectum, then shaving from retrocervical region is required.[9]
- In rectal endometriosis which has less than half of diameter involved, not penetrating the mucosa, discoid resection can be done.
- If the mucosal penetration is complete with endometriotic nodule, then we have to do rectal resection and reanastomosis using linear stapler.

CONCLUSION

The aim of surgery in endometriosis is fertility preservation and prevention of recurrence and adhesion. Hence, deep endometriosis requires a thorough preoperative investigation and appropriate surgical planning. It is imperative to perform a careful, thorough, and critical preoperative analysis of the clinical data and the findings of the various imaging techniques. Meticulous planning of appropriate treatment is imperative to avoid surgical complications. Thereafter, the surgical approach for bowel, bladder, ureter, etc. will depend on the symptoms of the patient and the extent of invasion of each organ involved by the disease. The surgical team must be multidisciplinary, composed of gynecologists, urologists, and colorectal surgeons. All visible and palpable lesions of the disease must be excised for the patient to reap real benefits. The concept of "one shot surgery" is the best option.

REFERENCES

1. Shaw RW. Treatment of endometriosis. Lancet. 1992;340(8830):1267-71.
2. Jain N, Sareen S, Kanawa S et al. Jain point. Jain point: A new safe portal for laparoscopic entry in previous surgery cases. J Hum Reprod Sci. 2016;9(1):9-17.
3. Koninckx PR, Martin DC. Deep endometriosis: a consequence of infiltration or retraction or possibly adenomyosis externa? Fertil Steril. 1992;58:924-8.

4. Oliveria MAP, Raymundo TS, Soares LC, et al. How to use CA-125 more effectively in the diagnosis of deep endometriosis. Biomed Res Int. 2017;2017:9857196.
5. Koninckx PR, Muyldermans M, Meuleman C, et al. CA 125 in the management of endometriosis. Eur J Obstet Gynecol Reprod Biol. 1993;49(1-2):109-13.
6. Reich H, McGlynn F, Salvat J. Laparoscopic treatment of cul-de-sac obliteration secondary to retrocervical deep fibrotic endometriosis. J Reprod Med. 1991;36(7):516-22.
7. Wolthuis AM, Meuleman C, Tomassetti C, et al. Bowel endometriosis: colorectal surgeon's perspective in a multidisciplinary surgical team. World J Gastroenterol. 2014; 20(42):15616-23.
8. Abrao MS, Petraglia F, Falcone T, et al. Deep endometriosis infiltrating the recto-sigmoid: critical factors to consider before management. Hum Reprod Update. 2015;21(3): 329-39.
9. Roman H, Drissa SM, Marty N et al. Rectal shaving for deep endometriosis infiltrating the rectum: a 5-year continuous retrospective series. Am Soc Reprod Med. 2016; 106(6):1438-45.

CHAPTER 9

Rectosigmoid Endometriosis/Deep Infiltrative Endometriosis

Parul Kotdawala, Santwan B Mehta

INTRODUCTION

Endometriosis is a progressive and benign estrogen-dependent disease defined by the presence of endometrial tissue (glands and stroma) outside the uterine cavity.[1] There are three types of endometriosis: (1) Peritoneal or surface endometriosis, (2) Endometrioma, and (3) Deeply infiltrating endometriosis (DIE). Each of these may occur alone or coexist with other forms.[2] DIE is a specific entity, unique in terms of origin, location, histology, and clinical symptoms.

The deep invasive endometriosis is defined as a form of endometriosis with rectovaginal lesions as well as infiltrative forms that involve vital structures like bowel, ureters, and bladder. DIE is a lesion that penetrates into the retroperitoneal space and/or the wall of the pelvic organs to a depth of at least 5 mm.[3] Peritoneal, ovarian, and deep endometriosis may be diverse manifestations of a disease with a single origin.[4] Deep lesions are considered very active and are strongly associated with pelvic pain symptoms.[3] Hormonal medicines induce temporary quiescence of active deep lesions and may be useful in selected cases, however, in most cases of severely infiltrating disease, a surgery is the final solution.[4]

PREVALENCE

The prevalence of endometriosis and the DIE seems to have increased over past 2 decades. This may be due to a growing awareness and also a quicker referral. Studies report that 15–30% of women with endometriosis will have deep infiltrating disease as well, although this might vary according to the referral patterns.[5,6] Mostly a deep endometriosis is associated with other forms of the disease like superficial implants, endometriotic ovarian cysts, and/or pelvic adhesions. In one study, an isolated deep endometriosis in absence of other endometriotic lesions was present in only 6.5%.[7] Urinary tract endometriosis is a rare entity, affecting approximately 1–2% of all cases of endometriosis,[8] while ureteral involvement is seen in 0.1–0.4% of all cases of endometriosis.[9]

HISTOGENESIS

The mechanism by which endometriosis develops is still subject of research, but four major theories have been proposed for the development of endometriosis:

1. *Retrograde menstruation (Samson's theory)*—it suggests that retrograde flow of menstrual blood into the abdominal cavity through the fallopian tubes carries and deposits endometrial cells in peritoneal cavity.[10] Implantation is due to favorable hormonal environment and to a failure of immune mechanisms to eliminate these cells.[11,12]
2. *Coelomic metaplasia theory*—the germinal epithelia of the ovary, endometrium, and peritoneum all originate from the same totipotential coelomic epithelium. The metaplasia theory postulates that these totipotential cells are transformed by repeated exposure to hormonal or inflammatory stimuli into endometrial tissues.[13] This might explain the development of endometriotic lesions in unusual locations as seen in cases of DIE.
3. *Vascular dissemination theory*—endometrial cells can be transported to extrauterine sites by blood vessels or the lymphatic channels or by contamination of the pelvis or abdominal wall incision if the uterine cavity is surgically entered. Retroperitoneal endometriosis is hypothesized to arise from lymph vascular spread.

4. *Autoimmune theory*—alterations in cellular immunity can facilitate the successful implantation of translocated endometrial cells. Animal research has shown that compared with control subjects, monkeys with spontaneous endometriosis had a lowered cell-mediated response to autologous endometrial tissue. This decreased cytotoxic response to endometrial cells that may lead to development of endometriotic implants.

Promoting factors—clinical and laboratory studies support the concept that endometriosis is an estrogen-dependent condition. Estradiol concentrations >60 pg/mL are felt necessary for proliferation of endometriotic lesions. Growth factors can originate from the peritoneal environment to stimulate endometrial development. Menstrual effluent contains factors that induce alterations in the peritoneal mesothelium, facilitating adhesion of endometrial cells. Attachment of endometrial cells is enhanced by induction of adhesion molecules and their receptors and the overexpression of matrix metalloproteinases and plasminogen activators. These factors ensure local destruction of the extracellular matrix.

In summary, no single theory explains all cases of endometriosis, although the direct implantation mechanism seems the likely cause for most disease locations. While a combination of all theories may explain the development of DIE lesions.

HISTOLOGY

Deeply infiltrating endometriosis lesions are histologically composed of scanty endometrial glands and stroma, but with extensive fibrosis. Myofibroblast (contractile nonmuscle cells) play a crucial role in development of such fibrosis. Infiltration by endometrial glands and stroma leads to activation of such myofibroblasts. When activated, myofibroblasts display increased proliferation and hyperplasia of surrounding smooth muscles and fibrous tissue, resulting in nodule formation. As DIE is predominantly composed of fibrotic tissue, it has been suggested that it should be called deep fibrotic endometriosis.[14-16]

LOCATION

Deeply infiltrating endometriosis implants are located in specific locations, primarily in the posterior cul-de-sac area.[14,17] DIE may also involve the intestinal system and the urinary system. Posterior DIE can involve uterosacral ligaments,[18] torus uterinus (also known as carina of uterus—retrocervical area of uterus where uterosacral ligaments join together),[19] the posterior vaginal wall, and the anterior rectal wall.[17,20] The most common sites for DIE are the rectovaginal space and the rectosigmoid, with the majority of women being found to have disease in these areas.[21] Out of all cases of DIE, the uterosacral ligaments are involved in 69.2% cases, vagina is involved in 14.5% cases, intestinal system is involved in 9.9% cases, and bladder is involved in 6.4% cases.[17]

TYPES

Intestinal Deeply Infiltrating Endometriosis

Intestinal DIE is defined as a lesion infiltrating the bowel, at least up to the muscular layer, and usually this is the rectosigmoid colon.[17] The inflammation triggered by bleeding intraperitoneal endometriotic papules in the most dependent portion of the pouch of Douglas may result in adhesions between the adjacent peritoneal surfaces of the anterior rectal wall and posterior vaginal fornix, with subsequent infiltration of the muscular layers of both organs.[4]

Symptoms that should arouse suspicion of colorectal involvement include constipation alternating with diarrhea, rectal pain, tenesmus, dyspareunia, dyschezia, and dysmenorrhea. Cyclical rectal bleeding is present in one-third of women with rectosigmoid involvement. Clinical obstruction occurs only in 1% cases.[22,23]

Bladder Endometriosis

Endometriosis of bladder is defined as infiltration of muscularis propria of the urinary bladder.[17] Adenomyofibrohyperplasia is found at the site of infiltration and can lead to painful, ineffective bladder contractions, as well as to microcirculatory disturbances in the urothelium, with resulting micro- or macrohematuria.[8,24]

Ureteric Endometriosis

Ureteral involvement is seen in 0.1–0.4% of all cases of endometriosis.[9] Endometriosis of the ureter can be either extrinsic or intrinsic type.[25] In the extrinsic type, the ureter is compressed by the shrinkage of endometriosis tissue that encompasses it on the outside; this is typically seen in cases of bilateral ovarian endometriosis. The most common site of involvement is the distal third of ureter, near the region of the ovarian fossa. The left ureter is more commonly affected.

Intrinsic ureteric endometriosis is rarer and infiltrates multiple layers of the ureter. Extrinsic type presents four times more frequently than the intrinsic type.[26] Regardless of the type, its manifestations range from nonspecific pelvic pain to flank pain, renal obstruction (usually unilateral), and asymptomatic hydronephrosis, with loss of function of the affected kidney(s).

CLASSIFICATION

It is essential to take the location of the deeply infiltrating endometriotic lesions into account because where pelvic pain is concerned, the success of the surgical operation depends on how radical the surgical removal is.[27] A classification system for DIE lesions based on the anatomic distributions of the lesions for the appropriate surgical management had been suggested by Chapron C et al.[17]

- A: Anterior DIE:
  - A1: Bladder.
- P: Posterior DIE:
  - P1: Uterosacral ligament
  - P2: Vagina
  - P3: Intestine.

Subclassification of retroperitoneal lesions by locations [precisely defined with transrectal ultrasonography (USG) and magnetic resonance imaging (MRI)]:

- *Rectovaginal septum lesions (type I)*—these lesions are generally small and account for 10% of all DIE. They are situated under the peritoneal fold of pouch of Douglas and are not connected to the cervix.
- *Posterior wall fornix lesions (type II)*—these account for 65% of all DIE and are supposed to be arising from the posterior wall of fornix, extending to the rectovaginal septum. When very small, they may not reach up to the rectovaginal septum or rectal wall.
- *Hourglass-shaped lesions (type III)*—these account for the remaining 25% and appear to be a combination of types I and II. Generally, they are large (>3 cm), with higher possibility of rectal involvement (Figs. 1A to C).[28]

CLINICAL FEATURES

Deeply infiltrating endometriosis is associated with chronic pelvic pain (CPP), dysmenorrhea, dyspareunia, dyschezia, urinary symptoms, and infertility. Women with DIE suffer from the most severe painful symptoms.[3] DIE is a distinct entity and it has the ability to infiltrate neighboring tissues.[14,29] This characteristic of DIE leads implants to compress or infiltrate the subperitoneal nerve fibers, the reason for the severity of symptoms.[30]

Prevalence of different clinical features were studied by Bellelis P et al. in 892 DIE cases and they suggested that 56.8% patients were having CPP, 54.7% had deep dyspareunia, 48.3% had cyclical intestinal complaints, 28.4% had incapacitating dysmenorrhea, and 11.7% had cyclical urinary complaints. Important thing to note here was that only 3.7% patients had cyclical intestinal symptoms (bleeding and/or pain on defecation during the menstrual period) as their chief complaint. A possible explanation for the low rate of intestinal symptoms may be the difficulty in

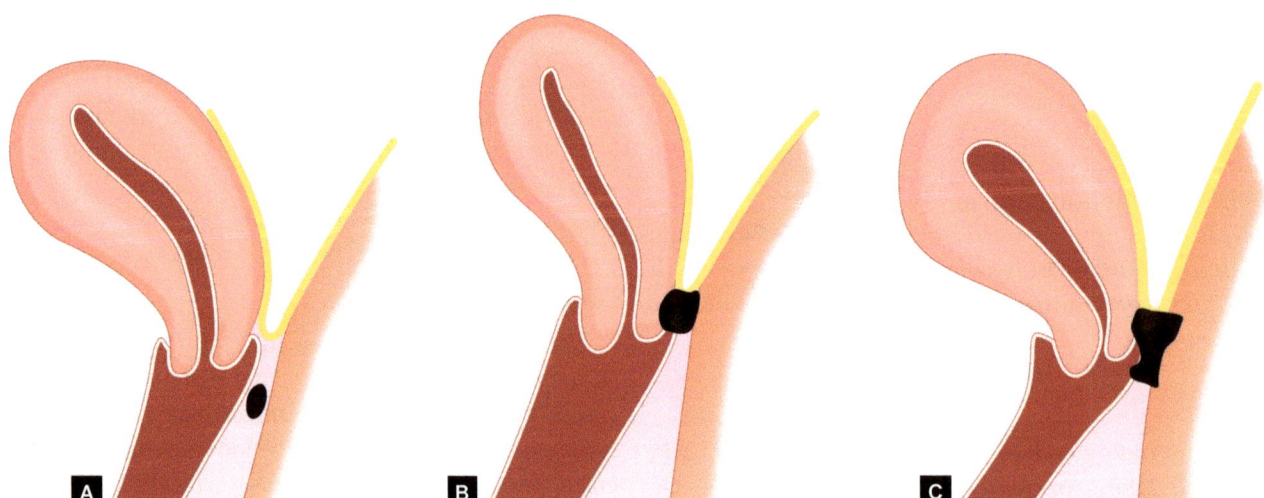

Figs. 1A to C: Classification of retroperitoneal deeply infiltrating endometriosis (DIE) lesions. Red spot—DIE lesion. (A) Left—type I—rectovaginal (RV) septum lesions (implants of RV septum 10%); (B) Center—type II—posterior wall fornix lesions (retroforniceal implants 65%); and (C) Right—type III—hourglass-shaped lesions (hourglass-shaped implants 25%).

distinguishing blood in feces from menstrual bleeding.[31] Another study (Gernot et al.—200 cases of DIE) showed dysmenorrhea 77.5%, dyspareunia 34.5%, dyschezia 14.5%, dysuria 2%, and CPP 22%.[32]

Relationship between different types of pelvic pain and specific locations of DIE was studied by Fauconnier et al. in 255 women.[33] Deep dyspareunia was correlated with involvement of the uterosacral ligament, painful defecation with the vagina, noncyclic pelvic pain with the bowel, lower urinary tract symptoms with the bladder, and gastrointestinal (GI) symptoms with the bowel and the vagina. In most cases, the pain is of the mechanical and provoked type—mobilization of the organs affected by DIE lesions triggers or aggravates the pain. Severe dysmenorrhea was not correlated with any DIE location, but was correlated with adhesions in the pouch of Douglas.[6] Dysmenorrhea could be due to cyclic recurrent microbleeding within the lesions and the consequent inflammation.[34,35] There is a direct relationship between the severity of dysmenorrhea and the presence of a rectal or vaginal infiltration by the posterior DIE and extensiveness of adnexal adhesion.[36] There is a significant correlation observed between dyschezia and posterior DIE. A positive correlation is seen between severity of dyschezia and lesion diameter and rectovaginal endometriosis, but not with anterior rectal wall involvement.[37]

Urinary tract disease may manifest as hydronephrosis caused by ureteral obstruction or as a submucosal lesion within the bladder or ureter. Psychological distress, depressive mood alterations, and/or clinically relevant depression or anxiety disorders are observed in >60% women with endometriosis.[38] Hence, a comprehensive clinical history is useful to identify patients at risk for endometriosis and to locate the disease.

DIAGNOSIS

Clinical Examination

Deep endometriosis should be suspected in all women having severe hypogastric pain, especially dysmenorrhea, deep dyspareunia, severe chronic pain, and dyschezia. Most pathognomonic signs are severe dyschezia, menstrual blood on stools, menstrual diarrhea, severe menstrual mictalgia (recurrent cystitis in premenstrual period), and radiation of pain to the perineum.[39]

The accuracy of clinical diagnosis is very limited, unless the nodule is seen on vaginal examination, or is palpated by rectal examination. Even a larger nodule (>3 cm in diameter) could be diagnosed in only 50% cases before 20 years. This may improve with experience and awareness.[40] For a smaller lesion, the diagnostic accuracy is poorer.

A palpable nodule, thickened area or a palpable cystic expansion on uterosacral ligaments, vagina, rectovaginal space, pouch of Douglas, the rectosigmoid, and the posterior wall of bladder are strong indicators of DIE.[41] A bimanual vaginal examination (one finger in vagina and one in rectum) can assess the rectovaginal space better. A clinical examination during menstruation is more reliable.[40]

Imaging Techniques

Several imaging studies have been used to preoperatively evaluate the DIE lesions, including transvaginal ultrasound (TVS), MRI of pelvis, and transrectal ultrasound (TRUS).[42-48] In addition to the diagnosis of DIE, the aim of preoperative imaging is to completely map all the deep implants, especially those affecting the digestive and/or urinary tract.[49]

In the specific case of the intestinal DIE, the preoperative imaging should give us following information:[43-45]
- Size of the lesion
- Depth of bowel wall infiltration
- Distance between intestinal DIE lesion and anal verge
- Percentage of intestinal circumference affected
- Presence of multifocal/multicentric intestinal DIE lesions.

Transvaginal Ultrasound

The clinical pelvic examination should be routinely combined with TVS in order to enhance diagnostic accuracy in all cases of endometriosis. A TVS is the first strategic tool for preoperative mapping of lesions and surgical planning.[41,47,50,51] Various specific evaluation techniques are proposed (rectal aqueous contrast, bowel preparations with laxatives, and vaginal injection of gel) to enhance the accuracy of imaging, but till date they remain inconclusive.[52]

The diagnostic value of TVS for noninvasive, presurgical detection of bowel endometriosis was checked in a large data pool and it was concluded that TVS with or without the use of prior bowel preparation is an accurate test for noninvasive, presurgical detection of DIE of the rectosigmoid.[41] Although the use of three-dimensional (3D) TVS has increased recently, an analysis of sensitivity and specificity of 3D TVS for a diagnosis of DIE in specific sites does not show any striking improvement in comparison to the conventional two-dimensional (2D) TVS.[53,54]

Hudelist G recommends a specific method of performing TVS to achieve adequate visualization of the affected organs. "First the transducer should be introduced into the posterior vaginal fornix and then it should be withdrawn backward to assess the pouch of Douglas, uterosacral ligaments, and the vagina wall. Following this, the probe should be advanced for visualization of the uterus and the adnexal regions in the sagittal and horizontal planes. In addition to this, bladder wall and paracervical areas (ureteral involvement) should also be visualized. Finally, the probe should be moved upward to achieve full visualization of the rectosigmoid wall layers, i.e. rectal muscle layer as well as rectal submucosa/mucosa (MUC) up to a level of 3–4 cm above the uterine fundus".[32,41] DIE is identified as hypoechoic, sometimes poorly delimited areas, roughly round, infiltrating the organ wall or location, and may occasionally contain hyperechoic foci.[55] The patients might complain of deep pain, when the transductor is pressed against an endometriotic focus.[56]

Endometriosis of the bladder was suspected in the presence of a paracervical lesion on TVS.[57] Since ureteral obstruction by DIE can lead to hydronephrosis, one should suspect involvement of ureter. As evolves into insidious renal failure, a urinary tract ultrasound scan, followed by specific tests for renal function are in order.

Rectal evaluation: Normally on TVS, rectal serosal tissue is not visualized as it is quite thin (0.5 mm) but rectal smooth muscle appears as a regular, hypoechogenic layer (2 mm thick) followed by a hyperechogenic line (1–2 mm) corresponding to the rectal submucosa and mucosa. If endometriotic infiltration is confined to serosal/smooth muscle (S/M) layer, it may appear as presence of hypoechogenic mass distorting the rectal smooth muscle with presence of a continuous hyperechogenic line corresponding to the intact mucosa. If rectal submucosa and mucosa are also infiltrated by the endometriosis, then there would be presence of a hypoechogenic mass only, within the rectal wall with complete absence of hyperechogenic line.[32,55,57-59] Bowel involvement is frequently multifocal, and the rectosigmoid colon is the most commonly affected area.[60] Intestinal evaluation is extremely important for the surgical approach and planning, since the number of lesions and the depth of invasion would decide the composition of surgical team, the equipment required, and the specific surgical technique.

Based on current data, it seems that involvement of the smooth muscle layer can be accurately determined by TVS in a large majority of patients with suspected DIE, but appears to be of little clinical value in detecting the infiltration of all rectal wall layers, i.e. infiltration of mucosal/submucosal layer.

Transrectal Ultrasonography

Transrectal USG with high-frequency probes has been recommended for detection of endometriosis in rectal, rectovaginal, uterosacral, or rectosigmoid locations.[61,62] Despite the fact that high-frequency (HF) sonography has poor penetration, the main advantage with this is that it provides a reliable means to diagnose any infiltration of the bowel wall.[63-65] Preliminary results show that rectal HF sonography appears to perform better than MRI for diagnosis of bowel wall infiltration.

Magnetic Resonance Imaging

Ultrasound gives equivocal results in some cases of rectovaginal or bladder endometriosis. MRI is quite useful to accurately predict the DIE in such cases.[66-68] MRI provides an advantage of the possibility of making a complete survey of anterior and posterior compartments of the pelvis at one time.[69] MRI is less operator dependent and can provide information about lesions at higher levels up to the sigmoid. Due to artifacts related to rectal content, deep rectal involvement is difficult to describe by the MRI, but phased-array coils, endovaginal coils, and rectal contrast enema may help to achieve better result.[70]

In conclusion, deep endometriosis is suspected or diagnosed clinically and the clinical suspicion can be confirmed by USG or MRI.

MANAGEMENT

General Principles

As endometriosis manifests differently in individual patients, it has a highly variable clinical course. The treatment should be designed according to the patient's personal needs rather than an arbitrary protocol.[71] This is best achieved by detailed discussion with the patient. DIE cases do not respond much to pharmacotherapy, and hence a surgery is the mainstay treatment, and laparoscopic approach is the gold standard for this.

Completeness of surgery with removal of all endometriosis (R0 resection) should be the goal, but evidence that endometriosis surgery needs to be 100% complete is lacking, and there are suggestions that opposite might be true. It is suggested, therefore, that deep endometriosis surgery should be visually complete and one can be less aggressive surgically.[39]

Chapron C et al. had suggested a classification system for DIE lesions based on anatomic distributions of the lesions for the appropriate surgical management.[17]

DIE Classification for Surgical Procedures

Classification of DIE	
DIE classification	Operative procedure
A: Anterior DIE	
A1: Bladder	Laparoscopic partial cystectomy
P: Posterior DIE	
P1: Uterosacral ligament	Laparoscopic resection of USL
P2: Vagina	Laparoscopic-assisted vaginal resection of DIE infiltrating posterior fornix
P3: Intestine	Solely intestinal
Without vaginal infiltration (V–)	Intestinal resection by laparoscopy/laparotomy
With vaginal infiltration (V+)	Laparoscopic-assisted vaginal intestinal resection or exeresis by laparotomy
Multiple intestinal location	Intestinal resection by laparotomy

(DIE: deeply infiltrating endometriosis; USL: uterosacral ligament)

Endometriosis of the Bladder

The primary treatment for symptomatic endometriosis of the bladder is a surgery,[8,25] and the surgeon's experience determines if this is best done via laparoscopy or laparotomy.[8,28] The infiltrated portion of the bladder should be dissected free from the cervicoisthmic junction till a visible disease-free vesicouterine space is reached. Now a partial vesical resection is performed to remove the endometriotic tissue.[8] After excising the endometriotic tissue, bladder wall is closed in two layers and bladder is catheterized for 7–10 days postoperatively. The most serious complication of this operation is neurogenic bladder, which may require long-term catheterization.

Endometriosis of the Ureter

In patients with ureteric endometriosis, the first step is to free the ureter from its surrounding tissue (ureterolysis) along its whole length. In addition to this, if there is intrinsic involvement of ureter is present, the involved segment should be resected followed by end-to-end anastomosis or direct ureteric implantation into the bladder. The peritoneum overlying the ureter, if involved, must be excised or vaporized. Periureteral vessels and retroperitoneal nerves must remain intact to prevent complications.[25]

Intestinal Deeply Infiltrating Endometriosis

The most common areas of intestinal involvement are the rectum and rectosigmoid colon. There are two important basic characteristics of intestinal DIE: (1) Multifocality and (2) Multicentricity. The multifocality (suggesting single disease with surrounding spread) is defined as the presence of other lesions within a 2-cm area to the main DIE lesion and the multicentricity (possibly multiple diseases) is defined as the separation of other lesions beyond 2 cm from the main DIE lesion. They are noted in 62% and 38% of surgical specimens, respectively.[72] These characteristics often decide the type of surgery in cases of intestinal DIE. Resection of the lesion is necessary as most of these lesions are fibrotic and usually unresponsive to hormonal therapy. These resection procedures to treat rectosigmoid DIE lesions can be divided mainly in two modes of surgery: (1) Conservative and (2) Radical.

Conservative surgery means the resection of the intestinal DIE implant. It is indicated for the lesions less than 2 cm in size or when the lesions involve less than one-third of the bowel circumference. Usually, the lesions are resected by the rectal shaving technique.[73-76] Shaving may be performed either completely or partially in the bowel wall when DIE lesions involve the rectal wall up to the muscular layer. In cases of the large lesions that encroach on the mucosa, full-thickness excision of involved bowel can be undertaken either by disk excision of small, isolated lesions or by segmental resection for larger lesions.[73,77,78] The anastomosis can be sutured with a continuous single layer of absorbable monofilament suture or created with surgical staples. The risk of rectovaginal fistula may be reduced by performing a defunctioning stoma.[79,80] Mucosal preservation is difficult and occasionally the rectal cavity might get opened during the procedure, which may be repaired by primary closure. A "partial shaving" is an emerging thought with recent advent of many young women with DIE. These women, having fertility issues also due to the DIE, may be treated with partial shaving, without going deeper into muscularis layers. They are then taken for assisted reproductive technology (ART) procedures soon after the surgery, and are allowed to complete the childbearing. They may be operated again for full excision, if symptoms of DIE persist or recur.

Radical surgery means resection of bowel segment affected by the endometriosis followed by primary colorectal anastomosis. It is indicated for the lesions of greater than 2–3 cm in size, for the lesions which cause bowel occlusion of greater than 50% of the circumference, when muscularis involvement of disease is greater than 7–8 cm and for multifocal/multicentric lesions.

The most appropriate surgical approach for rectosigmoid DIE still remains controversial.[81] The choice between conservative and radical treatment depends on the characteristics of the lesion, on preoperative imaging workup, surgeon's experience, and protocols.[82] As there is high rate of recurrence, more than 70% of women presenting with intestinal DIE end up segmental bowel resection.[81,83] Philippe et al. had suggested that women with a bowel occlusion of >50% or longer than 2–3 cm should be scheduled for elective bowel resection. All other women should undergo excision of the nodule.[40]

Some surgeons have also taken postoperative complications in account to decide the type of surgery and it has been found that the leakage rate and long-term consequences of bowel resection increase when the resection involves the lower part of the bowel. For sigmoid resection, leaks occur in <1% cases, almost without long-term problems, while for low rectal resections, leaks increase to 15% or more and carry a lifelong risk of dysfunction of bowel (30%), bladder (30%), and sexual problems (40%).[84] Therefore, it is suggested that for rectosigmoid and rectal nodules, one should attempt excision of bowel nodule, while for the sigmoid lesions one should be more liberal with bowel resections.[40]

There is a global trend toward minimally invasive approaches in the management of patients with intestinal DIE. Regardless of which technique is employed, one should keep in mind that endometriosis is a benign disease and that the main objective of the treatment is to improve the patient's quality of life. Prospective studies are still necessary to define which technique is the gold standard to manage intestinal DIE.

CONCLUSION

Deeply infiltrating endometriosis (DIE) is unique and specific entity of endometriosis, which is being detected more often, either due to rising incidence or perhaps because of increased awareness and finer imaging
techniques. It is associated with severe pelvic pain symptoms. A detailed history, careful pelvic examination and high quality imaging techniques (TVS, TRUS and MRI) can accurately diagnose the condition. Surgery remains the mainstay of treatment.

REFERENCES

1. Walter AJ, Hentz JG, Magtibay PM, et al. Endometriosis: correlation between histologic and visual findings at laparoscopy. Am J Obstet Gynecol. 2001;184:1407-11.
2. Donnez J, Nisolle M, Grandjean P, et al. The place of GnRH agonists in the treatment of endometriosis and fibroids by advanced endoscopic techniques. Br J Obstet Gynaecol. 1992;7:31-3.
3. Koninckx PR, Meuleman C, Demeyere S, et al. Suggestive evidence that pelvic endometriosis is a progressive disease, whereas deeply infiltrating endometriosis is associated with pelvic pain. Fertil Steril. 1991;55:759-65.
4. Vercellini P, Frontino G, Pietropaolo G, et al. Deep endometriosis: definition, pathogenesis, and clinical management. J Am Assoc Gynecol Laparosc. 2004;11: 153-61.
5. Keckstein J, Ulrich U, Kandolf O, et al. Laparoscopic therapy of intestinal endometriosis and the ranking of drug treatment. Zentralbl Gynakol. 2003;125:259-66.
6. Fauconnier A, Chapron C. Endometriosis and pelvic pain: epidemiological evidence of the relationship and implications. Hum Reprod Update. 2005;11:595-606.
7. Somigliana E, Infantino M, Candiani M, et al. Association rate between deep peritoneal endometriosis and other forms of the disease: pathogenetic implications. Hum Reprod. 2004;19:168-71.
8. Donnez J, Squifflet J, Donnez O, et al. Bladder endometriosis. In: Donnez J (Ed). Atlas of Operative Laparoscopy and Hysteroscopy. United Kingdom: Informa UK Ltd.; 2007. pp. 85-91.
9. Donnez J, Jadoul P, Donnez O, et al. Laparoscopic excision of rectovaginal and retrocervical endometriotic lesions. In: Donnez J (Ed). Atlas of Operative Laparoscopy and Hysteroscopy. United Kingdom: Informa UK Ltd.; 2007. pp. 63-75.
10. Sampson JA. Perforating hemorrhagic cysts of the ovary, their importance and especially their relation to pelvic adenomas of endometrial type. Arch Surg. 1921;3:245-7.
11. Podgaec S, Abrao MS, Dias JA, et al. Endometriosis: an inflammatory disease with a Th2 immune response component. Hum Reprod. 2007;22:1373-9.
12. Podgaec S, Abrão MS, Aldrighi JM. Aspectoshormonais da endometriose. In: Aldrighi JM (Ed). Endocrinologiaginecológica—aspectoscontemporâneos. São Paulo: Atheneu; 2005. pp. 221-8.
13. Meyer R. Uber den staude der frage der adenomyosite-sadenomyoma in allgemeinen und adenomyonetitis-sarcomatosa. Zentralbl Gynakol. 1919; 36:745-59 (Article in German).

14. Cornillie FJ, Oosterlynck D, Lauweryns JM, et al. Deeply infiltrating pelvic endometriosis: histology and clinical significance. Fertil Steril. 1990;53:978-83.
15. Donnez J, Nisolle M, Casanas-Roux F, et al. Stereometric evaluation of peritoneal endometriosis and endometriotic nodules of the rectovaginal septum. Hum Reprod. 1996;11:224-8.
16. Bochaton-Piallat ML, Gabbiani G, Hinz B. The myofibroblast in wound healing and fibrosis: answered and unanswered questions. F1000Res. 2016;5:752-9.
17. Chapron C, Fauconnier A, Vieira M, et al. Anatomic distribution of deeply infiltrating endometriosis: Surgical implications and proposition for a classification. Hum Reprod. 2003;18:157-61.
18. Chapron C, Dubuisson JB. Laparoscopic treatment of deep endometriosis located on the uterosacral ligaments. Hum Reprod. 1996;11:868-73.
19. Kamina P. Anatomie GyneÂcologique et obsteÂtricale 4. Paris: Maloine SA; 1984. p. 298 (Article in French).
20. Martin DC, Batt RE. Retrocervical, retrovaginal pouch, and rectovaginal septum endometriosis. J Am Assoc Gynecol Laparosc. 2001;8:12-7.
21. Vercellini P, Trespidi L, De Giorgi O, et al. Endometriosis and pelvic pain: relation to disease stage and localization. Fertil Steril. 1996;65:299-304.
22. Wang G, Tokushige N, Russell P, et al. Hyperinnervation in intestinal deep infiltrating endometriosis. J Minim Invasive Gynecol. 2009;16:713-9.
23. Slack A, Child T, Lindsey I, et al. Urological and colorectal complications following surgery for rectovaginal endometriosis. BJOG. 2007;114:1278-82.
24. Granese R, Candiani M, Perino A, et al. Bladder endometriosis: laparoscopic treatment and follow-up. Eur J Obstet Gynecol Reprod Biol. 2008;140:114-7.
25. Pérez-Utrilla Pérez M, Aguilera Bazán A, Alonso Dorrego JM, et al. Urinary tract endometriosis: clinical, diagnostic, and therapeutic aspects. Urology. 2009;73:47-51.
26. Howard WJ, John AR. Endometriosis. In: Jones HW, Rock JA (Eds). Te Linde's Operative Gynecology, 11th edition. India: Wolters Kluwer; 2014. pp. 403-45.
27. Garry R. Laparoscopic excision of endometriosis: the treatment of choice. Br J Obstet Gynaecol. 1997;104:513-5.
28. Donnez J, Squifflet J. Laparoscopic excision of deep endometriosis. Obstet Gynecol Clin North Am. 2004;31:567-80.
29. Donnez J, Nisolle M, Smoes P, et al. Peritoneal endometriosis and "endometriotic" nodules of the rectovaginal septum are two different entities. Fertil Steril. 1996;66:362-8.
30. Anaf V, Simon P, El Nakadi I, et al. Relationship between endometriotic foci and nerves in rectovaginal endometriotic nodules. Hum Reprod. 2000;15:1744-50.
31. Bellelis P, Dias JA, Podgaec S, et al. Epidemiological and clinical aspects of pelvic endometriosis—a case series. Rev Assoc Med Bras (1992). 2010;56:467-71.
32. Gernot H, Frank T, Gerald R, et al. Can transvaginal sonography predict infiltration depth in patients with deep infiltrating endometriosis of the rectum? Hum Reprod. 2009;24:1012-7.
33. Arnaud F, Charles C, Jean BD, et al. Relation between pain symptoms and the anatomic location of deep infiltrating endometriosis. Fertil Steril. 2002;78:719-26.
34. Fauconnier A, Chapron C, Dubuisson JB. Brosens IA. Endometriosis—a disease because it is characterized by bleeding. Am J Obstet Gynecol. 1997;176:263-7.
35. Vercellini P, Cortesi I, Crosignani PG. Progestins for symptomatic endometriosis: a critical analysis of the evidence. Fertil Steril. 1997;68:393-401.
36. Chapron C, Fauconnier A, Dubuisson JB, et al. Deep infiltrating endometriosis: relation between severity of dysmenorrhoea and extent of disease. Hum Reprod. 2003;18:760-6.
37. Seracchioli R, Mabrouk M, Guerrini M, et al. Dyschezia and posterior deep infiltrating endometriosis: analysis of 360 cases. J Minim Invasive Gynecol. 2008;15:695-9.
38. Halis G, Mechsner S, Ebert AD. The diagnosis and treatment of deep infiltrating endometriosis. Dtsch Arztebl Int. 2010;107:446-55.
39. Koninckx PR, Ussia A, Adamyan, et al. Deep endometriosis: definition, diagnosis, and treatment. Fertil Steril. 2012;98:564-71.
40. Koninckx PR, Meuleman C, Oosterlynck D, et al. Diagnosis of deep endometriosis by clinical examination during menstruation and plasma CA-125 concentration. Fertil Steril. 1996;65:280-7.
41. Hudelist G, Ballard K, English J, et al. Transvaginal sonography vs. clinical examination in the preoperative diagnosis of deep infiltrating endometriosis. Ultrasound Obstet Gynecol. 2011;37:480-7.
42. Piketty M, Chopin N, Dousset B, et al. Preoperative work-up for patients with deeply infiltrating endometriosis: transvaginal ultrasonography must definitely be the first-line imaging examination. Hum Reprod. 2009;24:602-7.
43. Kondo W, Zomer MT, Pinto EP, et al. Deep infiltrating endometriosis: imaging features and laparoscopic correlation. J Endometr. 2011;3:197-212.
44. Goncalves MO, Podgaec S, Dias JA, et al. Transvaginal ultrasonography with bowel preparation is able to predict the number of lesions and rectosigmoid layers affected in cases of deep endometriosis, defining surgical strategy. Hum Reprod. 2010;25:665-71.

45. Chamié LP, Pereira RM, Zanatta A, et al. Transvaginal US after bowel preparation for deeply infiltrating endometriosis: protocol, imaging appearances, and laparoscopic correlation. Radiographics. 2010;30:1235-49.
46. Chassang M, Novellas S, Bloch-Marcotte C, et al. Utility of vaginal and rectal contrast medium in MRI for the detection of deep pelvic endometriosis. Eur Radiol. 2010;20:1003-10.
47. Abrao MS, Gonçalves MO, Dias JA, et al. Comparison between clinical examination, transvaginal sonography and magnetic resonance imaging for the diagnosis of deep endometriosis. Hum Reprod. 2007;22:3092-7.
48. Takeuchi H, Kuwatsuru R, Kitade M, et al. A novel technique using magnetic resonance imaging jelly for evaluation of rectovaginal endometriosis. Fertil Steril. 2005;83:442-7.
49. Kondo W, Branco AW, Trippia CH, et al. Retrocervical deep infiltrating endometriotic lesions larger than thirty millimeters are associated with an increased rate of ureteral involvement. J Minim Invasive Gynecol. 2013;20:100-3.
50. Hudelist G, Oberwinkler KH, Singer CF, et al. Combination of transvaginal sonography and clinical examination for preoperative diagnosis of pelvic endometriosis. Hum Reprod. 2009;24:1018-24.
51. Savelli L, Manuzzi L, Coe M, et al. Comparison of transvaginal sonography and double-contrast barium enema for diagnosing deep infiltrating endometriosis of the posterior compartment. Ultrasound Obstet Gynecol. 2011;38:466-71.
52. Ferreira MC, Carneiro MM. Ultrasonographic Aspects of Endometriosis. J Endometr. 2010;2:47-54.
53. Grasso RF, Di Giacomo V, Sedati P, et al. Diagnosis of deep infiltrating endometriosis: accuracy of magnetic resonance imaging and transvaginal 3D ultrasonography. Abdom Imaging. 2010;35:716-25.
54. Guerriero S, Alcázar JL, Ajossa S, et al. Three-dimensional sonographic characteristics of deep endometriosis. J Ultrasound Med. 2009;28:1061-6.
55. Koga K, Osuga Y, Yano T, et al. Characteristic images of deeply infiltrating rectosigmoid endometriosis on transvaginal and transrectal ultrasonography. Hum Reprod. 2003;18:1328-33.
56. Goncalves MO, Dias JA, Podgaec S, et al. Transvaginal ultrasound for diagnosis of deeply infiltrating endometriosis. Int J Gynecol Obstet. 2009;104:156-60.
57. Bazot M, Malzy P, Cortez A, et al. Accuracy of transvaginal sonography and rectal endoscopic sonography in the diagnosis of deep infiltrating endometriosis. Ultrasound Obstet Gynecol. 2007;30:994-1001.
58. Dessole S, Farina M, Rubattu G, et al. Sonovaginography is a new technique for assessing rectovaginal endometriosis. Fertil Steril. 2003;79:1023-7.
59. Menada MV, Remorgida V, Abbamonte LH, et al. Transvaginal ultrasonography combined with water-contrast in the rectum in the diagnosis of rectovaginal endometriosis infiltrating the bowel. Fertil Steril. 2008;89:699-700.
60. Chapron C, Chopin N, Borghese B, et al. Deeply infiltrating endometriosis: pathogenetic implications of the anatomical distribution. Hum Reprod. 2006;21:1839-45.
61. Roseau G, Dumontier I, Palazzo I, et al. Rectosigmoid endometriosis: endoscopic ultrasound features and clinical implications. Endoscopy. 2000;32:525-30.
62. Chapron C, Dubuisson JB. Management of deep endometriosis. Ann N Y Acad Sci. 2001;943:276-80.
63. Chapron C, Dumontier I, Dousset B, et al. Results and role of rectal endoscopic ultrasonography for patients with deep pelvic endometriosis. Hum Reprod. 1998;13:2266-70.
64. Fedele L, Bianchi S, Portuese A, et al. Transrectal ultrasonography in the assessment of rectovaginal endometriosis. Obstet Gynecol. 1998;91:444-8.
65. Schröder J, Löhnert M, Doniec JM, et al. Endoluminal ultrasound diagnosis and operative management of rectal endometriosis. Dis Colon Rectum. 1997;40:614-7.
66. European Society of Human Reproduction and Embryology (ESHRE). (2007). ESHRE Guideline for the Diagnosis and Treatment of Endometriosis. [online] Available from http://guidelines.endometriosis.org/concise-pain.html. [Last accessed October, 2019].
67. Stratton P, Winkel C, Premkumar A, et al. Diagnostic accuracy of laparoscopy, magnetic resonance imaging, and histopathologic examination for the detection of endometriosis. Fertil Steril. 2003;79:1078-85.
68. Benacerraf BR, Groszmann Y. Sonography should be the first imaging examination done to evaluate patients with suspected endometriosis. J Ultrasound Med. 2012;31:651-3.
69. Balleyguier C, Chapron C, Dubuisson JB, et al. Comparison of magnetic resonance imaging and transvaginal ultrasonography in diagnosing bladder endometriosis. J Am Assoc Gynecol Laparosc. 2002;9:15-23.
70. Kinkel K, Chapron C, Balleyguier C, et al. Magnetic resonance imaging characteristics of deep endometriosis. Hum Reprod. 1999;14:1080-6.
71. Vercellini P, Carmignani L, Rubino T, et al. Surgery for deep endometriosis: A pathogenesis-oriented approach. Gynecol Obstet Invest. 2009;68:88-103.
72. Kavallaris A, Kohler C, Kühne-Heid R, et al. Histopathological extent of rectal invasion by rectovaginal endometriosis. Hum Reprod. 2003;18:1323-7.
73. Kondo W, Zomer MT, Ribeiro R, et al. Laparoscopic treatment of intestinal deep infiltrating endometriosis by laparoscopy—technical aspects. Bras J Video Surg. 2012.
74. Kondo W, Bourdel N, Jardon K, et al. Comparison between standard and reverse laparoscopic techniques for rectovaginal endometriosis. Surg Endosc. 2011;25:2711-7.

75. Kondo W, Bourdel N, Zomer MT, et al. Surgery for deep infiltrating endometriosis: technique and rationale. Front Biosci (Elite Ed). 2013;5:316-32.
76. Donnez J, Squifflet J. Complications, pregnancy and recurrence in a prospective series of 500 patients operated on by the shaving technique for deep rectovaginal endometriotic nodules. Hum Reprod. 2010;25:1949-58.
77. Crispi CP, Schor E, Oliveira MA, et al. Treaty of Gynecological Endoscopy: Cirurgia Minimally Invasive, 3rd edition. Rio de Janeiro: Revinter; 2012.
78. Woods RJ, Heriot AG, Chen FC. Anterior rectal wall excision for endometriosis using the circular stapler. ANZ J Surg. 2003;73:647-8.
79. Ruffo G, Sartori A, Crippa S, et al. Laparoscopic rectal resection for severe endometriosis of the mid and low rectum: technique and operative results. Surg Endosc. 2012;26:1035-40.
80. Choi DH, Hwang JK, Ko YT, et al. Risk factors for anastomotic leakage after laparoscopic rectal resection. J Korean Soc Coloproctol. 2010;26:265-73.
81. Meuleman C, Tomassetti C, D'Hoore A, et al. Surgical treatment of deeply infiltrating endometriosis with colorectal involvement. Hum Reprod Update. 2011;17: 311-26.
82. Roman H, Rozsnayi F, Puscasiu L, et al. Complications associated with two laparoscopic procedures used in the management of rectal endometriosis. JSLS. 2010;14:169-77.
83. De Cicco C, Corona R, Schonman R, et al. Bowel resection for deep endometriosis: a systematic review. BJOG. 2011; 118:285-91.
84. Ret Dávalos ML, De Cicco C, D'Hoore A, et al. Outcome after rectum or sigmoid resection: a review for gynecologists. J Minim Invasive Gynecol. 2007;14:33-8.

CHAPTER 10

Fertility Prevention and Endometriosis: What is the Status?

Surveen Ghumman

INTRODUCTION

Over the recent years the skill of fertility preservation technology has evolved to reach a level of acceptable results. It encompasses sperm and oocyte preservation. Ovarian tissue cryopreservation is still experimental although pregnancies have been reported. Till some time back these were indicated only to preserve fertility in cancer patients before they undergo radiotherapy and chemotherapy. Now indications have expanded to women who may be at risk of developing poor ovarian reserve because of nonmalignant causes. It is the category, under which women with endometriosis fall.

As endometriosis is a disease which adversely affects fertility, fertility preservation in its management may play a vital role. The endometrioma in the ovary may need a surgery and they may lead to substantial loss of normal healthy ovarian tissue. Women with endometriosis undergo repeated surgeries for pain and this may be damaging to the ovaries causing irreversible loss of ovarian follicles. However, surgery may be important specially in a fast-growing endometrioma as it could be malignant and a histological diagnosis is needed.

IMPACT OF ENDOMETRIOSIS ON OVARIAN RESERVE

Surgery does impact the ovarian reserve as has been seen in numerous studies. Somigliana et al. in 2012 did a meta-analysis which included 11 studies and found that there was statistically significant reduction of serum anti-Müllerian hormone (AMH) level after surgery.

The magnitude of the decline was more evident in women operated for bilateral endometriomas.[1]

Some amount of ovarian tissue is lost with stripping of the cyst wall. Ovarian tissue also gets damaged if cyst wall is ablated with electrocautery. It was seen that ovarian tissue was present in cyst wall of 65% of those who underwent laparoscopic stripping of cyst and 80% of those where this technique was done by laparotomy. This showed that laparoscopy may help in better dissection and less loss of ovarian tissue. However, when compared to simple cyst the incidence in simple cyst was only 31–40% showing that endometriosis is a more adherent and difficult cyst to take out and hence a real threat to the ovarian reserve exists when this cyst is operated on.[2]

The factors which determine the amount of loss of follicle is dependent on many factors like the use of electrocautery, amount of inflammation, number of pre-existing follicles, and whether endometrioma is bilateral. It is also related to how many times the surgery is done and the expertise of the surgeon. It has also been reported that extensive surgery like adhesiolysis done around ovary may impair the ovarian reserve even though ovary may not be touched. This may be because of interruption of ovarian vascularity. The tissue around the endometrioma shows a higher amount of fibrosis and lower density of follicles.[3-5]

In a recent study it was seen that serum AMH decreased significantly at the 6th month (61%) postoperatively. The AMH decrease was more in bilateral compared with unilateral endometriomas (67% vs. 57%, respectively). Basal AMH level was the only independent factor affecting the AMH decrease (odds ratio, 3.68).[6] The impact on ovarian reserve manifested after ovarian surgery as longer stimulation, higher follicle stimulating hormone (FSH) requirement and lower oocyte number, but fertilization, pregnancy, and implantation rates did not differ between the groups.[7,8]

COUNSELING FOR FERTILITY PRESERVATION IN ENDOMETRIOSIS

It is imperative to counsel these women that their fertility span is limited and give them their choices. A clear understanding of the success rates of the in vitro fertilization (IVF) cycle with frozen eggs must be given so that they can decide on number of cycles they would like to undergo. One should advise to ideally freeze 12–20 eggs. Often these women may be older with a lower AMH. Hence they have to be advised about multiple cycles to have enough eggs frozen for optimum IVF results. Counseling on age-related yield and IVF success rates in relation to endometriosis must be done.

In vitro fertilization outcomes in endometriosis: There are studies which show a poor outcome in IVF because of poor oocyte and embryo quality. However many studies have refuted these findings. In a recent study which included a total of 22,416 women it was concluded that although women with endometriosis generate fewer oocytes, fertilization rate is not impaired and the likelihood of achieving a live birth is also not affected.[9]

FACTORS TO BE CONSIDERED BEFORE FERTILITY PRESERVATION

Decisions must be taken keeping in view the age of the patient, severity of disease, ovarian reserve, and whether it is bilateral, progression of disease, and need for surgery. Fertility preservation is indicated not only in severe disease but women with mild disease and a low AMH should also be considered. It should also be contemplated in young women with a normal AMH, who still need to start a family.

OPTIONS OF FERTILITY PRESERVATION IN ENDOMETRIOSIS

Fertility Preserving Surgery

In women who have not completed their family it is important to perform an optimum fertility preserving surgery. Deep coagulation which can lead to permanent damage of cortex and blood vessels is to be avoided. Surgical techniques leading to minimal adhesions postoperatively should be used to prevent tubal block.[10]

Ablation and resection of cyst wall are the two acceptable options for removal of cyst. Simple aspiration or coagulation as a surgical therapy is unacceptable as it has a high recurrence rate.[11] An experienced surgeon with additional knowledge on reproductive medicine is important. Removal of cyst should be done with care not to damage surrounding healthy tissue. Bipolar cauterization can cause significant ovarian damage and should be avoided.[12]

Cases should be individualized avoiding surgery in small (less than 4 cm) endometriomas, women with low AMH levels or those with bilateral endometrioma. However surgeon's skill is important in these cases, so one cannot have a blanket rule.

In case of extensive endometriosis with dense adhesions it is difficult to do a fertility sparing surgery. These cases must definitely go for fertility preservation before surgery. Also, patients with bilateral endometriomas and those with a low AMH must have counseling for fertility preservation before surgery.

It must be kept in mind that all cases can have medium-term recurrence of lesions which was observed in 20% of the cases, and 25% of the women underwent repetitive surgery. Repeat surgery will lead to further decrease in ovarian reserve.[13]

Indications for Surgery before Oocyte Retrieval for Fertility Preservation

Very large endometriomas also cause difficulty in visualization and monitoring size of follicle by ultrasound becomes difficult. Surgery is indicated when there is difficulty in retrieving oocytes because endometrioma is obstructing the field, as this will prevent optimum retrieval of oocytes. Surgery will be needed before oocyte retrieval. Puncturing and draining the endomerioma is an option though it can lead to infection and abscess formation and is not recommended as a standard treatment.

Oocyte and Embryo Freezing

The oocyte freezing which was earlier experimental is a well-established treatment specially for those women without a partner who would like to preserve their fertility. For those who have a partner embryo freezing is preferred.

Does Ovarian Stimulation Increase Endometriosis or its Symptoms?

In a study conducted by D'Hooghe et al. with a 21-month follow-up, it was seen that those women who underwent IVF had lower recurrence rates (7%) than the overall study population.[14] Another study showed that after IVF there was no increase in symptoms, or in size and number of lesions. The number (%) of women reporting general improvement and worsening were 14 (22%) and 7 (11%), respectively.[15]

Hence it was concluded ovarian stimulation or IVF does not lead to disease progression in endometriosis.

Would Presence of Endometrioma Impact Egg Yield and Subsequent IVF Results?

There has been no evidence to suggest that removal of endometrioma improves the IVF cycle results or the egg yield. A meta-analysis by Laursen in 2017 showed no difference in live birth rates on comparison of conservative management and after surgery (OR: 0.87). Although the mean difference of antral follicle count was 2.09.[16] There are studies which show a lower egg yield but live birth rates remain the same.[9]

Risk of Oocyte Retrieval with Endometriosis

Since an invasive procedure takes place in the presence of collected blood, chances of abscess formation and pelvic inflammatory disease are much higher while doing an oocyte retrieval in these cases.[17] In case of accidental puncture a pelvic abscess may result. All these women must be counseled about this risk before start of treatment.

Specific Indications for Oocyte and Embryo Freezing

There are certain situations in which oocyte or embryo freezing must be recommended like those with an already compromised egg reserve (low AMH). These women will further reduce their AMH to near zero levels after surgery. Somigliana et al. stated that it should in particular be recommended for those with bilateral unoperated endometriomas and for those who previously had excision of unilateral endometriomas and require surgery for a contralateral recurrence.[17,18]

Ovarian Cortex Freezing

This requires the stripping out of the ovarian cortex which contains the primordial follicles. These follicles are relatively resistant to ischemia and can survive while tissue is cut into thin strips and frozen. However, this is not recommended in endometriosis as there is further loss of ovarian tissue in an already compromised ovary. In case cystectomy is done the wall of the cyst can be looked for in the ovarian tissue and the same can be cryopreserved. Carillo et al. in their review article stated clearly that a deliberate removal of normal cortical tissue should be viewed as a potential threat for ovarian reserve. The indication for such intervention is therefore not entirely clear and such option should be critically discussed in light of its potential risks and benefits in women with endometriosis.[19]

Cost-benefit Analysis of Fertility Preservation in Women with Endometriosis

Somigliana et al. have argued against fertility preservation for all women with endometriosis. The lack of any randomized controlled trials to evaluate the final outcome should be taken into account. They have stated that there is insufficient data for robust cost-utility analyses. Cost-benefit analysis becomes very important in a disease like endometriosis as it is relatively a common disease unlike cancer and there is a large group which would be required to undergo this treatment if it gets started as a norm. This would have huge financial and logistic implications as it is a costly treatment.

They recommended that more clinical data and in-depth economic analysis are essential prior to recommending its routine use.[1,18]

In conclusion, fertility preservation is an important option which should be offered to all women with endometriosis, specially those with a decreased AMH and bilateral endometriomas. For women who have not completed their family fertility sparing surgery done by an experienced surgeon is important as ovarian reserve is impacted if healthy ovarian tissue gets removed at cystectomy. Counseling for women going in for oocyte and embryo cryopreservation is important to explain success rates of IVF and the number of oocytes required to be retrieved for optimum results. Oocyte cryopreservation is a well-recognized procedure and no longer experimental. Ovarian tissue cryopreservation is still experimental although pregnancies have been reported. Despite justification for fertility preservation in endometriosis we still need to do a cost-benefit analysis and identify a population which would substantially benefit.

REFERENCES

1. Somigliana E, Berlanda N, Benaglia L, et al. Surgical excision of endometriomas and ovarian reserve: a systematic review on serum antimüllerian hormone level modifications. Fertil Steril. 2012;98(6):1531-8.
2. Alborzi S, Foroughinia L, Kumar PV, et al. A comparison of histopathologic findings of ovarian tissue inadvertently excised with endometrioma and other kinds of benign ovarian cyst in patients undergoing laparoscopy versus laparotomy. Fertil Steril. 2009;92(6):2004-7.

3. Kitajima M, Defrère S, Dolmans MM, et al. Endometriomas as a possible cause of reduced ovarian reserve in women with endometriosis. Fertil Steril. 2011;96(3):685-91.
4. Li CZ, Liu B, Wen ZQ, et al. The impact of electrocoagulation on ovarian reserve after laparoscopic excision of ovarian cysts: a prospective clinical study of 191 patients. Fertil Steril. 2009;92(4):1428-35.
5. Hirokawa W, Iwase A, Goto M, et al. The postoperative decline in serum anti-Mullerian hormone correlates with the bilaterality and severity of endometriosis. Hum Reprod. 2011;26(4):904-10.
6. Celik HG, Dogan E, Okyay E, et al. Effect of laparoscopic excision of endometriomas on ovarian reserve: serial changes in the serum antimüllerian hormone levels. Fertil Steril. 2012;97(6):1472-8.
7. Demirol A, Guven S, Baykal C, et al. Effect of endometrioma cystectomy on IVF outcome: a prospective randomized study. Reprod Biomed Online. 2006;12(5):639-43.
8. Benschop L, Farquhar C, van der Poel N, et al. Interventions for women with endometrioma prior to assisted reproductive technology. Cochrane Database Syst Rev. 2010;(11):CD008571.
9. González-Comadran M, Schwarze JE, Zegers-Hochschild F, et al. The impact of endometriosis on the outcome of Assisted Reproductive Technology. Reprod Biol Endocrinol. 2017;15(1):8.
10. Muzii L, Marana R, Angioli R, et al. Histologic analysis of specimens from laparoscopic endometrioma excision performed by different surgeons: does the surgeon matter? Fertil Steril. 2011;95(6):2116-9.
11. Practice Committee of the American Society for Reproductive Medicine. Endometriosis and infertility: a committee opinion. Fertil Steril. 2012;98(3):591-8.
12. Seyhan A, Ata B, Uncu G. The impact of endometriosis and its treatment on ovarian reserve. Semin Reprod Med. 2015;33(6):422-8.
13. Vercellini P, Crosignani PG, Abbiati A, et al. The effect of surgery for symptomatic endometriosis: the other side of the story. Hum Reprod Update. 2009;15(2):177-88.
14. D'Hooghe TM, Denys B, Spiessens C, et al. Is the endometriosis recurrence rate increased after ovarian hyperstimulation? Fertil Steril. 2006;86(2):283-90.
15. Benaglia L, Somigliana E, Santi G, et al. IVF and endometriosis-related symptom progression: insights from a prospective study. Hum Reprod. 2011;26(9):2368-72.
16. Brink Laursen J, Schroll JB, Macklon KT, et al. Surgery versus conservative management of endometriomas in subfertile women: A systematic review. Acta Obstet Gynecol Scand. 2017;96(6):727-35.
17. Elizur SE, Lebovitz O, Weintraub AY, et al. Pelvic inflammatory disease in women with endometriosis is more severe than in those without. J Obstet Gynaecol. 2014;54(2):162-5.
18. Somigliana E, Viganò P, Filippi F, et al. Fertility preservation in women with endometriosis: for all, for some, for none? Hum Reprod. 2015;30(6):1280-6.
19. Carrillo L, Seidman DS, Cittadini E, et al. The role of fertility preservation in patients with endometriosis. J Assist Reprod Genet. 2016;33(3):317-23.

CHAPTER 11

Scar Endometriosis—Preservation Strategies and Management

Pratik Tambe, Riddhi Desai

INTRODUCTION

Scar endometriosis is a relatively rare form of endometriosis that develops at the site of the surgical incision subsequent to obstetric or gynecological surgeries. It is also known as abdominal wall endometriosis, cutaneous endometriosis or endometrioma externa.[1] Even though the most common form of endometriosis is endopelvic endometriosis, where most of the endometrial deposits are found in the pelvis, which include the ovaries, the peritoneum, the uterosacral ligaments, the pouch of Douglas, and the rectovaginal septum. It may also rarely occur in extrapelvic locations, which may be found in up to 1% of the women with endometriosis.[2]

The various extrapelvic sites include most of the body cavities, as well as organs which include the lung, gallbladder, bowel, kidney, central nervous system, extremities, perineum, and the abdominal wall.[3,4] Any surgery that involves contact with endometrial tissue is at risk of scar endometriosis. Most commonly, it occurs in cesarean section, hysterectomy, episiotomy, laparotomy, and laparoscopic surgeries.[5,6]

INCIDENCE

The actual incidence is difficult to determine as it remains under diagnosed and under reported. The first case was reported by Meyer in 1903.[7] Since then, most of the literature available is in the form of case reports. There are however, only five studies that calculated the incidence rate in a study group of more than 3,000 women with cesarean sections each, with an average incidence rate of 0.15%.[8] Some of the recent literature report incidences ranging from 0.03% to 1% of all women undergoing any surgical procedure.[9]

This marked rise in incidence of scar endometriosis is due to the increase in frequency of cesarean section and laparoscopy. The incidence after hysterectomy is reported to be 1.08–2%, and 1% after mid-trimester abortion.[10] It may also be seen after surgical procedures like appendectomy, episiotomy, amniocentesis, and inguinal herniorrhaphy.[11] Studies have also reported that it can occur after laparoscopic gastric bypass and cholecystectomy.[12] The incidence of concomitant pelvic endometriosis with scar endometriosis has been reported to be 14.3–26%.[13]

PATHOPHYSIOLOGY

The pathophysiology is still not clear. Different theories for abdominal wall endometriosis have been described.[14,15]

- Most cases can be explained by iatrogenic dissemination of decidual tissue. The probable etiology is mechanical transplantation or direct implantation of viable endometrial cells into the scar during surgery which subsequently proliferate or induce metaplasia under the influence of estrogen. However, this does not explain the existence of endometriosis in the abdominal wall without any previous surgery.
- Sampson's theory postulated the implantation or retrograde menstruation hypothesis which states that endometrial tissue from the uterus is shed during menstruation and transported retrograde through the fallopian tubes, thereby gaining access to and implanting on pelvic structures.
- Coelomic metaplasia theory states that cells in the abdomen undergo metastasis induced by hormonal manipulation.
- Another theory suggests lymphatic or vascular dissemination.

CLINICAL DIAGNOSIS

Symptoms of endometriosis are frequently not recognized which results in delay in the diagnosis and therapy of the scar endometriosis. In most cases, women present to the clinic with symptoms months to years after a surgery. Usually, patients are referred to general surgeons and may sometimes be misdiagnosed.

The most common symptoms are:[16,17]

- Pain and swelling, which worsen during menstruation. Clinical examination may reveal a painful and palpable nodule with maximum tenderness over the scar during menstruation in a patient with a previous history of gynecological or obstetrical surgery. Biswas et al. reported fluctuation of swelling size after each menstrual cycle.
- Vague symptoms, such as abdominal pain, more often, colicky type on surgical site, are the most common symptoms.
- Hypertrophic and hyper pigmented scars due to hemosiderin deposits are seen.

However, in the largest reported series to date, only 20% of the patients exhibited these types of symptoms.[18] According to many studies, the time interval between surgery and presentation varied between 3 months and 10 years.[19]

RISK FACTORS[20]

Certain risk factors have been identified:

- There is a higher incidence in mid-trimester abortions which may be due to pluripotential capability of early decidua, resulting in cellular replication producing endometriomas.
- Early hysterotomy (less than 22 weeks)
- Cesarean section performed before spontaneous onset of labor
- Early hysterectomy
- Heavy menstrual flow
- Alcohol consumption.

DIAGNOSIS[21-23]

It is not an easy condition to diagnose, only half of them present with classical symptoms and may be confused with incision hernia, abscess, hematoma, lipoma, carcinoma (primary), granule, lymphoma, neuroma, cyst, abscess or soft tissue sarcoma. This results in a considerable delay in the diagnosis and initiation of treatment. A high index of suspicion is recommended with postoperative abdominal lump as well as in those where there is absence of classical symptoms. The presence of cyclical pain in an incision mass during menstruation is almost pathognomonic. Histopathological examination remains the gold standard for diagnosis of scar endometriosis. However, it is pertinent to use noninvasive diagnostic modalities before any surgical intervention.

There are various methods for diagnosis of scar endometriosis:

- Ultrasonography is a useful tool to detect scar endometriosis in an early stage. Preoperative imaging is valuable in detecting the extent of the disease and planning an accurate excision. However, ultrasound accuracy is reduced in obese patients. Early diagnosis is of importance since delayed diagnosis creates repair problems during surgery, the possible need of meshes and can cause deformities.
- Fine-needle aspiration cytology (FNAC) is a simple procedure with high specificity.
- MRI enables detection of very small lesions. It is superior to CT scan for detection of the planes between the muscle and subcutaneous tissue.
- Color Doppler may be useful when there is a large lesion on the abdominal wall.

HISTOPATHOLOGY[24]

Histological diagnosis of endometriosis is based on the identification of characteristic endometrial glands and associated stromal cells outside the cavum uteri and deposition of hemosiderin pigment. The abdominal wall endometriosis may show deposit in the dermis, subcutaneous tissue, rectus abdominis muscle, and rectus sheath. The excised tissue shows endometrial glands in cellular stoma. Enhanced mitotic figures are seen along with some RBC and chronic inflammatory cells.

TREATMENT

Management must be individualized according to the clinical presentation. Treatment is not required in an asymptomatic patient. Mainstay of treatment is always surgical excision in symptomatic cases. It is both diagnostic and curative. A wide local excision is preferred and if the defect is large can be repaired with a Polypropylene mesh.[25,26] Medical therapy with combined oral contraceptives (COCs), progestogens, androgens or gonadotropin-releasing hormone (GnRH) analogs gives reduction of the symptoms temporarily, with recurrence after cessation of the therapy.[27]

RECOMMENDATIONS FOR PREVENTION[28,29]

- Removing decidual tissue while closing the uterus and cleansing with normal saline has been described as a preventive measure.
- Use different mops and needles for different layers.
- Intraoperative contamination of the surrounding tissue with the endometrial cells is a situation that should be taken into account during operations in the pelvis. Therefore, sweeping the uterus with gauze during a cesarean delivery should be limited.
- It is recommended that the abdominal wound should be thoroughly cleaned, especially, around the corners.

Risk of Malignancy

Malignant changes in scar endometriosis are rare, less than 1%. It should be suspected in a long-standing case with recurrence.[30]

CONCLUSION

Scar endometriosis remains a diagnostic challenge. The question remains whether the actual incidence is as low as been stated in most of the current literature or that the complication is underestimated. An increasing trend in the incidence justifies more attention to the diagnosis and requires research into pathophysiology and prevention. To improve the detection rate of scar endometriosis, a high index of suspicion, more attention to medical history, and physical examination are mandatory. In view of increasing cesarean and hysterectomy rates, it is of utmost importance to form and implement best practice guidelines for any surgery, to prevent the transplantation of endometrial tissue over the site of scar.

REFERENCES

1. Ozturk A, Kaya C, Bozkurtoglu H, et al. Scar endometrioma: An uncommon yet easily treated condition. J Reprod Med. 2016;61(5-6):249-53.
2. Kodandapani S, Pai MV, Mathew M. Umbilical laparoscopic scar endometriosis. J Hum Reprod Sci. 2011;4(3):150-2.
3. Bergqvist A. Extragenital endometriosis. A review. Eur J Surg. 1992;158(1):7-12.
4. Wolf GC, Singh KB. Cesarean scar endometriosis: a review. Obstet Gynecol Surv. 1989;44(2):89-95.
5. Steck WD, Helwig EB. Cutaneous endometriosis. JAMA. 1965;191:167-70.
6. Albrecht LE, Tron V, Rivers JK. Cutaneous endometriosis. Int J Dermatol. 1995;34(4):261-2.
7. Wyrens RG, Randall LM. Endometriosis in scars. Am J Surg. 1942;56:397-403.
8. Adriaanse B, Natté R, Hellebrekers B. Scar endometriosis after a caesarean section: a perhaps underestimated complication. Gynecol Surg. 2013;10(4):279-84.
9. Tatli F, Gozeneli O, Uyanikoglu H, et al. The clinical characteristics and surgical approach of scar endometriosis: A case series of 14 women. Bosn J Basic Med Sci. 2018;18(3):275-8.
10. Singh KK, Lessells AM, Adam DJ, et al. Presentation of endometriosis to general surgeons: a 10-year experience. Br J Surg. 1995;82(10):1349-51.
11. Blanco RG, Perithivel VS, Shah AK, et al. Abdominal wall endometriomas. Am J Surg. 2003;185(6):596-8.
12. Applebaum GD, Iwanczyk L, Balingit PB. Endometrioma of the abdominal wall masquerading as hernia. Am J Emerg Med. 2004;22(7):621-2.
13. Nirula R, Greaney GC. Incisional endometriosis: an underappreciated diagnosis in general surgery. J Am Coll Surg. 2000;190(4):404-7.
14. Pathan Z, Rao R, Dinesh U, et al. Scar endometriosis. J Cytol. 2010;27(3):106-8.
15. Ideyi SC, Schein M, Niazi M, et al. Spontaneous endometriosis of the abdominal wall. Dig Surg. 2003;20(3):246-8.
16. Leite GK, Carvalho LF, Korkes H, et al. Scar endometrioma following obstetric surgical incisions: retrospective study on 33 cases and review of the literature. Sao Paulo Med J. 2009;127(5):270-7.
17. Khoo JJ. Scar endometriosis presenting as an acute abdomen: a case report. Aust N Z J Obstet Gynaecol. 2003;43(2):164-5.
18. Modi R, Jain M, Polara J. Scar endometriosis: A rare case report. Int J Med Sci Public Health. 2017;6(55):974-6.
19. Seydel AS, Sickel JZ, Warner ED, et al. Extrapelvic endometriosis: diagnosis and treatment. Am J Surg. 1996;171(2):239.
20. Nominato NS, Prates LF, Lauar I, et al. Caesarean section greatly increases risk of scar endometriosis. Eur J Obstet Gynecol Reprod Biol. 2010;152(1):83-5.
21. Chauhan V, Pujani M, Singh K, et al. Scar endometriosis with rudimentary horn: An unusual and elucidative report of a case diagnosed on Histopathology and immunohistochemistry. J Mid-life Health. 2017;8:196-9.
22. Tangirala S, Pratha A, Isukapalli V, et al. Scar endometriosis: a clinical rarity. IAIM. 2015;2(5):147-51.
23. Danielpour PJ, Layke JC, Durie N, et al. Scar endometriosis—a rare cause for a painful scar: A case report and review of the literature. Can J Plast Surg. 2010;18(1):19-20.
24. Pachori G, Sharma R, Sunaria RK, et al. Scar endometriosis: Diagnosis by fine needle aspiration. J Cytol. 2015;32(1):65-7.

25. Catalina-Fernández I, López-Presa D, Sáenz-Santamaria J. Fine needle aspiration cytology in cutaneous and subcutaneous endometriosis. Acta Cytol. 2007;51(3):380-4.
26. Schoelefield HJ, Sajjad Y, Morgan PR. Cutaneous endometriosis and its association with caesarean section and gynaecological procedures. J Obstet Gynaecol. 2002;22(5):553-4.
27. Rivlin ME, Das SK, Patel RB, et al. Leuprolide acetate in the management of cesarean scar endometriosis. Obstet Gynecol. 1995;85(5 Pt 2):838-9.
28. Bektas H, Bilsel Y, Sari YS, et al. Abdominal wall endometrioma; a 10-year experience and brief review of the literature. J Surg Res. 2010;164:e77-81.
29. Wasfie T, Gomez E, Seon S, et al. Abdominal wall endometrioma after cesarean section: a preventable complication. Int Surg. 2002;87(3):175-7.
30. Agarwal N, Subramanian A. Endometriosis. morphology, clinical presentations and molecular pathology. J Lab Physicians. 2010;2(1):1-9.

CHAPTER 12

Endometriosis and Infertility

Rohan Palshetkar, Nandita Palshetkar

INTRODUCTION

Endometriosis is a long-term, recurrent, debilitating disease experienced by 5–10% women. It remains an everlasting challenge to the healthcare providers, one of the important reasons being a delay in its diagnosis.[1]

Endometriosis affects 1 in 10 women of reproductive age worldwide. The prevalence of endometriosis as reported is between 2% and 10% in the normal women, 20–50%[2,3] in the infertile population and more than 60%[4] in women with chronic pelvic pain and dysmenorrhea. Maximum incidence is seen in the age group of 25–30 years.

Endometriosis is characterized classically by the presence of endometrial glands and stroma outside the endometrial cavity in ectopic locations like the pelvic peritoneum, ovaries, and retrocervical septum.[5,6]

The monthly fecundity rate (MFR) in a normal couple in the reproductive age group is around 30% in the first three cycles and <4% after 1 year. In endometriosis, MFR is reduced to 2–10% per month. Even minimal endometriosis may present with severe infertility.

FACTORS CAUSING INFERTILITY IN ENDOMETRIOSIS

- Ovulatory dysfunction
- Immunological alterations
- Peritoneal factors
- Sperm inactivation—phagocytosis by macrophages
- Interference with implantation—endometrial dysfunction
- Interference with coital function—dyspareunia
- *Mechanical factors*:
  - Anatomical distortion of tubes
  - Altered tubal motility
  - Interference with ovum pick up

Peritubal adhesions: The adverse effect of pelvic endometriosis on uterine cavity is seen not only before conception but even after, resulting in deep placentation and subsequently predisposing the woman to preeclampsia and antepartum hemorrhage in pregnancy.[7]

CLINICAL FEATURES[8]

Clinical features have been shown in Box 1.

DIAGNOSIS OF ENDOMETRIOSIS

Clinical examination must be performed in all women suspected to have endometriosis, although vaginal examination may not be appropriate for adolescents and women without any prior sexual intercourse. In some cases, rectal examination may be helpful especially when rectal endometriosis or ovarian endometrioma is suspected.

When painful induration and/or rectovaginal wall nodules are felt and visible in the posterior vaginal fornix on clinical examination, the diagnosis of deep endometriosis may be considered.[9]

When adnexal masses are detected on clinical examination, the diagnosis of ovarian endometriosis may be strongly considered.

BOX 1: Clinical features of endometriosis.

The Guideline Development Group (GDG) recommends that the diagnosis of endometriosis should be considered in a women with any of the below:
- Gynecological symptoms like dysmenorrhea, chronic pelvic pain, deep dyspareunia, infertility, and fatigue.
- Nongynecological cyclical symptoms like dyschezia, dysuria, hematuria, shoulder pain or rectal bleeding in a woman of reproductive age.

Table 1: Typical and atypical features of endometriomas.	
Typical USG features of endometrioma	Atypical features of endometriomas
• Oval mass • Hypoechoic content • Hyperechogenic wall • Absence of papillae	• Septa • Inhomogenous content • Irregular internal wall • Papillary projections

(USG: ultrasonography)

Sometimes even in presence of endometriosis, the clinical examination is normal.[10] Transvaginal sonography is a very good modality to diagnose or exclude ovarian endometrioma[11] and rectal endometriosis, but in the latter, a highly experienced operator is required (Tables 1 and 2).[1]

A monolateral, unilocular image < 5 cm in the ovary, without septa or papillae with very sparse vascularization independent of its content's density has very little possibility of being malignant.

- Doppler ultrasound is of great help in the differential diagnosis, as most endometriomas show the typical peripheral vascularization whereas other show the "hilus sign" described by Kurjak, which is the presence of vessels between the cyst capsule and the ovarian parenchyma.
- Three-dimensional (3D) ultrasonography (USG) to diagnose rectovaginal endometriosis is not well established. Magnetic resonance imaging (MRI) is useful in diagnosis of extraovarian endometriosis.[12]
- Biomarkers in the endometrial tissue or follicles or menstrual blood and/or (cancer antigen-125) should not be used to diagnosis endometriosis.[13]
- Laparoscopy along with histological confirmation of endometriotic glands and/or stroma is the gold standard for diagnosis.

MANAGEMENT OPTIONS

- Medical
- Surgical
- Combined medical and surgical
- Intrauterine insemination/in vitro fertilization/intracytoplasmic sperm injection (IUI/IVF/ICSI)
- Oocyte freezing.

Medical Treatment

Currently all the available treatment options for endometriosis are suppressive rather than curative. So, there is temporary relief of symptoms during the treatment and on discontinuation, recurrence is the rule. The most common indication for medical treatment is pain. The current treatment options for endometriosis associated pain are contraceptive in nature by blocking the hypothalamic-pituitary-ovarian (HPO) axis.

In women with endometriosis associated with pain, nonsteroidal anti-inflammatory drugs (NSAIDs) appear to be the only medical option. In a systematic review of three clinical trials[14] pretreatment with a gonadotropin-releasing hormone (GnRH) agonist for 3–6 months before IVF or ICSI in endometriosis improved the clinical pregnancy rate fourfold.

With aggressive disease, medical therapy may fail and consequently a large proportion of women may require multidisciplinary surgeries (Table 3).

Dienogest

Dienogest (DNG) has been described in Table 4.

Gonadotropin-releasing Hormone Agonists

Gonadotropin-releasing hormone agonist has been described in Table 5.

Table 2: Differential diagnosis of endometriotic cyst and ovarian endometrioma.					
Differential diagnosis of endometriotic cyst					Differential diagnosis of ovarian endometrioma
	Endometrioma	Corpus luteum	Cystadenoma	Dermoid	• Cystadenoma • Dermoid cyst • Hemorrhagic cyst • Luteinized unruptured follicle • Corpus luteum
Septa	Infrequent	No	Frequent	Infrequent	
Inhomogenous content	Infrequent	Frequent	Rare	Frequent	
Posterior reinforcement	No	No	No	Frequent	
Hyperechogenic dots	Frequent	No	No	No	

Table 3: Food and Drug Administration (FDA) and non-FDA-approved medical therapies.

Medical therapy[15]

FDA-approved therapies:	Non-FDA-approved therapies:

• Three GnRH agonists:
  1. Leuprolide
  2. Goserelin
  3. Nafarelin
• Two progestins:
  1. Depot medroxyprogesterone acetate 150 mg intramuscular (IM) every 3 months. This may cause decrease in bone density with long-term use
  2. Norethindrone acetate (oral) is the only oral progestin approved by the FDA. Dose—5 mg/day orally for 2 weeks, then increased by 2.5 mg/day every 2 weeks till 15 mg is reached for total 6–9 months
• Danazol:
  – Antiestrogenic with weak androgen agonistic properties
  – Causes anovulation and suppression of menses by inhibiting gonadotropins, immunomodulatory action and inhibition of cell proliferation
  – Category X drug
	• Ovulation suppressing agents:
	  – Combined hormonal contraceptives usually recommended as first-line therapy in adolescents with endometriosis and in those without contraindication to hormonal treatment
	• Progestins:
	  – Oral medroxyprogesterone acetate 20–30 mg/day for 6 months
	  – Dienogest (2 mg/day)
	• GnRH antagonists:
	  – Cetrorelix acetate 3 mg subcutaneous weekly over an 8-week period
	  – Elagolix (oral)
	• Anti-inflammatory agents:
	  – NSAIDs—according to a Cochrane review although NSAIDs are used as a first-line treatment in suspected endometriosis, there is little evidence for significant reduction in pain
	  – No one NSAID is more effective than the other. Along with OLPs, usually given as first-line therapy.
	  – COX-2 inhibitors (rofecoxib)—inhibits PG synthesis—withdrawn from the US market due to cardiovascular risk
	  – Peroxisome proliferator—activated receptor gamma agonists (PPAR-γ; rosiglitazone, pioglitazone)
	  – Pentoxifylline—not commonly used
	  – Antioxidants—role is speculative
	• Agents acting on endometriotic deposits directly:
	  – Aromatase inhibitors (inhibition of estrogen formation in ovarian granulosa cells and also in endometriotic deposits)
	    ♦ Letrozole, anastrozole—concern is formation of functional cysts due to superovulation
	  – Levonorgestrel intrauterine device (LNG-IUD)
	    ♦ Progesterone receptor antagonists or selective progesterone receptor modulators—mifepristone
	  – Selective estrogen receptor modulator (SERM)—raloxifene
	  – Statins—e.g. simvastatin
	• Immunomodulators—e.g. infliximab, etanercept
	• Angiogenesis inhibitors—cabergoline, quinagolide
	• Gestrinone
	• Valproic acid
	• Melatonin
	• Phytoestrogens—isoflavones

(COX: cyclooxygenase; GnRH: gonadotropin-releasing hormone; NSAIDs: nonsteroidal anti-inflammatory drugs; OLPs: oral lichen planus; PG: peptidoglycan)

Table 4: Dienogest (DNG).

Type	Fourth generation selective progestin steroid
Route	Oral
Mechanism of action (MOA)	Anovulation, antiproliferation, inhibition of cytokine secretion from endometrial stromal cells
Additional effects	Antiandrogenic. Profound local effects on local endometriotic implants with minimal impact on metabolic parameters
Dose	2 mg daily is usually recommended
Comparison with other drugs	• When compared with norethisterone acetate (NETA) at 2.5 mg, DNG at 2 mg gave comparable symptomatic relief and health-related quality of life (QOL).[16] Due to high cost of DNG, it can be given in patients who do not tolerate NETA • In a recent systematic review of eight randomized controlled trials (RCTs), comparing DNG with gonadotropin-releasing hormone (GnRH) agonist which included 1,273 women with symptomatic endometriosis, DNG was superior to placebo but equivalent to GnRH agonists in controlling pain symptom in endometriosis[17]
Pharmacokinetics	Oral absorption rapid with 90% bioavailability, exclusively bound to albumin (90%), $t_{1/2}$ 10 hours reacting state concentration after 2 days of administration, metabolism in liver[18]
Uses	In superficial and deep infiltrating endometriosis with or without visceral involvement
Safety profile	Side effects though not common are mild-to-moderate headache, breast discomfort, depressed mood, acne, nausea, vaginal bleeding In a pooled analysis from four European RCTs, DNG at 2 mg dose was well-tolerated and safe for up to 65 weeks[19]

Endometriosis and Infertility

Table 5: Gonadotropin-releasing hormone (GnRH) agonists.

Route	Intramuscular. Subcutaneous or intranasal
Drug available	Leuprolide acetate (parenteral) Nafarelin acetate (intranasal) Goserelin acetate (subcutaneous) Triptorelin
Manufacturing	Substitution of L-amino acid by D-amino acid at position 6 of the native GnRH, thus making it resistant to degradation and giving a longer half-life
Mechanism of action (MOA)	Administration of GnRH agonist ↓ ↑ Initial pituitary flare (FSH and LH) (This may exacerbate endometriosis symptoms. This can be blunted by aromatase inhibitors for first 7–10 days of treatment or giving GnRH agonist in the luteal phase of the cycle)[20] ↓ Downregulation of pituitary GnRH receptor ↓ Decrease in FSH & LH ↓ Ovarian suppression→↓ ↓ E_2 and P within 1 month of GnRH use, the E_2 levels will be in the menopausal range
Effects	Direct effects on endometriotic implants
Efficacy	Second or third-line medical treatment after combined oral contraceptives (COCs) and progestin for endometriosis associated pain. Pain relief is between 50% and 90%. Combined surgical and medical treatment with GnRH agonists has the lowest recurrence rate and highest cure rate[21-23]
Add-back HT	• GnRH agonist therapy can lead to hypoestrogenic side effects like hot flushes, mood swings, vaginal dryness, decreased libido, bone loss, and headache. Therefore add-back HT is used to treat these side effects and prevent any long-term sequelae. Only progesterone or a combination of estrogen or progesterone may be used. This does not affect the efficiency of GnRH agonist • Most commonly used is NETA 5 mg daily as add-back agent and is approved by the US-FDA • Typically, GnRH agonist is used for 3–6 months and could be extended to 1 year • Add-back therapy should be started along with GnRH agonist therapy as this will reduce the vasomotor symptoms and pressure bone density. According to "estrogen threshold hypothesis", E_2 concentration of 30–45 pg/mL is required to maintain bone density • Also patients must be instructed to take adequate calcium and vitamin D along with HT • In those who cannot use HT as add-back they may benefit from herbal remedies, selective serotonin reuptake inhibitors (SSRIs) and serotonin or norepinephrine reuptake inhibitors • Alternatively, dose of GnRH agonist may be reduced or interval between doses may be increased[24,25]
Doses	Leuprolide acetate — 3.75 mg once a month or 11.25 mg every 3 months
	Nafarelin acetate — 1 spray (200 µg) in the morning and evening Total 400 µg/day for 6 months
	Goserelin acetate — 3.6 mg every 4 weeks for 6 months in ≥18 years women
	Triptorelin — 3.75 mg every 4 weeks

(E_2: estradiol; FDA: Food and Drug Administration; FSH: follicle-stimulating hormone; HT: hormone therapy; LH: luteinizing hormone; NETA: norethisterone acetate; P: progesterone)

In extrapelvic and deep infiltrating endometriosis (DIE): DIE involves the uterosacral ligaments, rectovaginal septum, bowel, and ureters or urinary bladder. GnRH agonists are usually the first-line agents as they suppress ovarian hormone production and inhibit the growth of ectopic endometrial growth.[26]

Surgical Treatment

Surgery may be the first-line management in:[27]
- Highly symptomatic women
- Those with a normal ovarian reserve
- Unilateral and large cysts
- Those suspicious of malignancy.

After an initial surgery for infertility, performing any additional surgery will not increase the fecundability and such patients should be better subjected to assisted reproductive technology (ART).

Combined Medical and Surgical Treatment

Although theoretically beneficial, there is no evidence to support that combined medical and surgical therapy improves fertility. On the contrary, it may unnecessarily delay any further fertility therapy.

Assisted Reproductive Technology

Certain patients' profiles may benefit from proceeding directly to IVF which are:
- Asymptomatic women
- Women with advanced reproductive age
- Bilateral endometriomas
- Prior surgical treatment as surgery may have a detrimental effect on the ovarian reserve and delay the initiation of treatment.

Ovarian Endometrioma[28,29]

Endometrioma is a pseudocyst originating from the ectopic endometrial tissue in the ovary and progresses by invaginating in to the ovarian cortex.[30] It may be symptomatic or asymptomatic and is found in 17–44% of women with endometriosis. It can be diagnosed reliably by transvaginal USG.

Current medical treatment does not resolve an endometrioma. Also, surgical removal will diminish the ovarian reserve which has been seen in a systematic review.[31]

Risks and Benefits of Surgical Therapy of Endometrioma versus Expectant Management

Surgery

Risks and benefits of surgery have been shown in Table 6.

Expectant Management

Risks and benefits of expectant management have been shown in Table 7.

Endometrioma treated surgically has a high recurrence rate and using this option for women undergoing IVF has been challenged.[33] It has been reported that due to the technical difficulty involved in removal of endometriomas as they are usually adherent to the normal ovarian tissue, tissue rim containing primordial follicles is removed in more than 50% endometriomas.[34] This results in diminished ovarian reserve after its surgical removal.

European Society of Human Reproduction and Embryology (ESHRE) guidelines state that there is no evidence that cystectomy before starting ART has any improvement in the pregnancy rate.

CONCLUSION

Endometriosis is quite a common disease in women with infertility. Early diagnosis and appropriate management is crucial in managing early onset endometriosis. One must consider the diagnosis of endometriosis even when the clinical examination is normal in the presence of symptoms. An adnexal mass with diffuse low level internal echoes and absence of neoplastic features is highly suggestive of an endometrioma. While formulating a treatment plan for a particular patient, all factors like age, duration of infertility, symptoms, and stage of endometriosis must be considered. In infertile women having endometriosis, hormonal treatment like contraceptives, progestins, GnRH analogs or danazol for suppressing ovarian function must

Table 6: Advantages and disadvantages of surgical therapy.

Advantages	Disadvantages
• Facilitates access to oocyte retrieval • Symptom relief • Rules out malignancy • Minimizes risk of cyst complications	• Reduction of ovarian reserve and chances of ovarian failure as in 13% patients, normal tissue may be destroyed[32] • Increased gonadotropin requirement • Surgical risks • Postoperative adhesions • Recurrence

Table 7: Advantages and disadvantages of expectant management.

Advantages	Disadvantages
• No surgical risk • Increased oocyte retrieval • Ovarian reserve maintained • May require comparatively lower dose of gonadotropins • No delay in starting assisted reproductive technology	• Pain • Small chance of pelvic infection following oocyte retrieval • No tissue available for histopathological diagnosis • Cyst rupture • Difficulties in accessing the ovaries at the time of oocyte retrieval • Contamination of follicular fluid • Accelerated progression of the disease

not be prescribed to improve fertility. In minimal or mild endometriosis, medical management does not improve spontaneous pregnancy rates, but surgery is beneficial. The presence of an endometrioma does not appear to adversely affect IVF outcomes, and its surgical excision does not appear to improve IVF outcomes. There is no evidence that endometriosis cause cancer, nor there is an overall increase, but in these women incidence of some cancers like that of ovary and non-Hodgkins' lymphoma is slightly more. As compared to no management, ART improves the pregnancy rates. Women with endometriosis may benefit from a combination of medical, surgical, and ART therapy. Individualization of care is important.

REFERENCES

1. Hudelist G, Fritzer N, Thomas A, et al. Diagnostic delay for endometriosis in Austria and Germany: causes and possible consequences. Hum Reprod. 2012;27:3412-6.
2. Giudice LC, Kao L. Endometriosis. Lancet. 2004;364:1789-99.
3. Ilangavan K, Kalu E. High prevalence of endometriosis in infertile women with normal ovulation and normospermic partners [letter]. Fertil Steril. 2010;93:e10.
4. Guo SW, Wang Y. The prevalence of endometriosis in women with chronic pelvic pain. Gynecol Obstet Invest. 2006;62:121-30.
5. Burney RO, Giudice LC. Pathogenesis and pathophysiology of endometriosis. Fertil Steril. 2012;98:511-9.
6. Batt RE, Martin DC, Odunsi K. Endometriosis of the retrocervical septum is proposed to replace the anatomically incorrect term endometriosis of the rectovaginal septum. Hum Reprod. 2014;29:2603-5.
7. Brosens I, Brosens JJ, Fusi L, et al. Risks of adverse pregnancy outcome in endometriosis. Fertil Steril. 2012;98:30-5.
8. Dunselman GA, Vermeulen N, Becker C, et al. ESHRE guideline: management of women with endometriosis. Hum Reprod. 2014;29:400-12.
9. Bazot M, Lafont C, Rouzier R, et al. Diagnostic accuracy of physical examination, transvaginal sonography, rectal endoscopic sonography, and magnetic resonance imaging to diagnose deep infiltrating endometriosis. Fertil Steril. 2009;92:1825-33.
10. Chapron C, Dubuisson JB, Pansini V, et al. Routine clinical examination is not sufficient for diagnosing and locating deeply infiltrating endometriosis. J Am Assoc Gynecol Laparosc. 2002;9:115-9.
11. Moore J, Copley S, Morris J, et al. A systematic review of the accuracy of ultrasound in the diagnosis of endometriosis. Ultrasound Obstet Gynecol. 2002;20:630-4.
12. Pascual MA, Guerriero S, Hereter L, et al. Diagnosis of endometriosis of the rectovaginal septum using introital three-dimensional ultrasonography. Fertil Steril. 2010;94:2761-5.
13. May KE, Conduit-Hulbert SA, Villar J, et al. Peripheral biomarkers of endometriosis: a systematic review. Hum Reprod Update. 2010;16:651-74.
14. Sallam HN, Garcia Velasco JA, Dias S, et al. Long-term pituitary down-regulation before in vitro fertilization (IVF) for women with endometriosis. Cochrane Database Syst Rev. 2006:CD004635.
15. Quaas AM, Weedin EA, Hansen KR, et al. On-label and off-label drug use in the treatment of endometriosis. Fertil Steril. 2015;103:612-25.
16. Vercellini P, Bracco B, Mosconi P, et al. Norethindrone acetate or dienogest for the treatment of symptomatic endometriosis: a before and after study. Fertil Steril. 2016;105:734-43.
17. Andres Mde P, Lopes LA, Baracat EC, et al. Dienogest in the treatment of endometriosis: systematic review. Arch Gynecol Obstet. 2015;292:523-9.
18. Bińkowska M, Woroń J. Progestogens in menopausal hormone therapy. Prz Menopauzalny. 2015;14:134-43.
19. Strowitzki T, Faustmann T, Gerlinger C, et al. Safety and tolerability of dienogest in endometriosis: pooled analysis from the European clinical study program. Int J Womens Health. 2015;7:393-401.
20. Bedaiwy MA, Mousa NA, Casper RF. Aromatase inhibitors prevent the estrogen rise associated with the flare effect of gonadotropins in patients treated with GnRH agonists. Fertil Steril. 2009;91:1574-7.
21. Alkatout I, Mettler L, Beteta C, et al. Combined surgical and hormone therapy for endometriosis is the most effective treatment: prospective, randomized, controlled trial. J Minim Invasive Gynecol. 2013;20:473-81.
22. Song JH, Lu H, Zhang J, et al. [Clinical study on the effectiveness and safety of combined laparoscopy and gonadotropin-releasing hormone agonist in the treatment of endometriosis]. Zhonghua Fu Chan Ke Za Zhi. 2013;48:584-8.
23. Harada M, Osuga Y, Izumi G, et al. Dienogest, a new conservative strategy for extragenital endometriosis: a pilot study. Gynecol Endocrinol. 2011;27:717-20.
24. Uemura T, Shirasu K, Katagiri N, et al. Low dose GnRH agonist therapy for the management of endometriosis. J Obstet Gynaecol Res. 1999;25:295-301.
25. Kang JL, Wang XX, Nie ML, et al. Efficacy of gonadotropin-releasing hormone agonist and an extended-interval dosing regimen in the treatment of patients with adenomyosis and endometriosis. Gynecol Obstet Invest. 2009;69:73-7.

26. Korom S, Canyurt H, Missbach A, et al. Catamenial pneumothorax revisited: clinical approach and systematic review of the literature. J Thorac Cardiovasc Surg. 2004;128:502-8.
27. Jayaprakasan K, Becker C, Mittal M. The Effect of Surgery for Endometriomas on Fertility: Scientific Impact Paper No. 55. BJOG. 2018;125:e19-28.
28. Vercellini P, Fedele L, Aimi G, et al. Reproductive performance, pain recurrence and disease relapse after conservative surgical treatment for endometriosis: the predictive value of the current classification system. Hum Reprod. 2006;21:2679-85.
29. Gelbaya TA, Nardo LG. Evidence-based management of endometrioma. Reprod Biomed Online. 2011;23:15-24.
30. Hachisuga T, Kawarabayashi T. Histopathological analysis of laparoscopically treated ovarian endometriotic cysts with special reference to loss of follicles. Hum. Reprod. 2002;17:432-5.
31. Raffi F, Metwally M, Amer S. The impact of excision of ovarian endometrioma on ovarian reserve: a systematic review and meta-analysis. J Clin Endocrinol Metab. 2012;97:3146-54.
32. Almog B, Sheizaf B, Shalom-Paz E, et al. Effects of excision of ovarian endometrioma on the antral follicle count and collected oocytes for in vitro fertilization. Fertil Steril. 2010;94:2340-2.
33. Garcia-Velasco JA, Somigliana E. Management of endometriomas in women requiring IVF: to touch or not to touch. Hum Reprod. 2009;24:496-501.
34. Muzii L, Bianchi A, Croce C, et al. Laparoscopic excision of ovarian cysts: is the stripping technique a tissue-sparing procedure? Fertil Steril. 2002;77:609-14.

CHAPTER 13

Surgery before In Vitro Fertilization: What is the Evidence and Recommendations?

Fessy Louis T, Parvathy T

INTRODUCTION

Endometriosis is commonly associated with infertility and subfertility. The various proposed reasons for endometriosis causing infertility include activity of various inflammatory mediators, poor ovarian reserve, access to oocyte retrieval difficult in severe endometriosis, poor quality oocytes, and reduced implantation rates. The role of medical and surgical treatment options in treating the symptom severity has limited role when infertility aspect is concerned. The disease severity has a negative correlation between the pregnancy rates in endometriosis.[1] These factors can be overcome by the use of assisted reproductive techniques.

Most of the cases of endometriosis being associated with pelvic pain, which can be managed medically. Even it being an insidious disease, surgical management may be the necessary part of treatment algorithm. With the advancement in the field of preoperative imaging, laparoscopy is rarely needed for diagnosis of endometriosis. When planning for surgery, the ideal goal should be a therapeutic and effective surgical intervention based on preoperative evaluation.

Nowadays, the most important role of laparoscopy related to endometriosis is in the management of pain. The role for surgery in woman with endometriosis due to pain might be indicated in patients who are not willing for surgery or those with contraindication for medical therapy, any acute surgical events, case of deep endometriosis, in concomitant management with other gynecologic disorders, and those with fertility with associated pain.

The laparoscopy may be considered in infertile patients in those having hydrosalpinges undergoing assisted reproductive technology (ART), the management of ovarian endometrioma may be considered in special situations on request from a patient as an alternative to in vitro fertilization (IVF).[2] Surgery should be undertaken with special care with keeping in mind the potential risk of future fertility.

Several studies have reported that patients with ovarian endometriomas had a decreased response to ovarian stimulation during IVF treatment cycle. The management of ovarian endometrioma with respect to infertility is based on the size of endometriotic cyst as concluding from different articles. In those with endometriotic cyst size less than 3 cm, it has been advised that they do not need any preliminary measures and can start with IVF cycle. In those having endometriotic cyst measuring 3–5 cm, gonadotropin-releasing hormone (GnRH) agonist needs to be given at least 3–6 months prior to IVF treatment.[3] Those having endometriotic cyst measuring more than 5 cm or any endocyst interfering with oocyte retrieval needs to undergo either cyst aspiration or ovarian cystectomy prior to oocyte retrieval.

Broadly, the role of surgery for endometriosis prior to IVF can be considered in the following conditions:
- Mild-to-moderate endometriosis
- Improving access for oocyte retrieval
- Treating hydrosalpinx to improve IVF outcome
- Ovarian endometrioma and suspicion of concomitant malignancy
- Concomitant management of disease
- Patient deferring IVF due to personal, cultural, or religious reason
- If the patient opt for surgery or not willing for ART.

MILD-TO-MODERATE ENDOMETRIOSIS

Endometriosis is going to negatively affect fertility in a number of ways. The various reasons for negative effect on fertility include chronic inflammatory state produced by the disease condition per se, the pelvic adhesions disrupting the anatomy interfering with oocyte and embryo transport, and diminished ovarian reserve produced by endometriosis. Theoretically, the surgical management should improve the atmosphere for successful conception. As per the recent Cochrane review as put forward by Duffy et al. the laparoscopic management in case of mild and moderate endometriosis increase the rates of live birth and ongoing pregnancy. The success rate is below 50% for IVF in case of embryo transfer in presence of endometriosis. In some cases, surgical management of endometriosis may improve the fecundity rate and helps the couple to conceive often without IVF. The primary reason proposed for negative result due to endometriosis in IVF is mainly due to defective endometrial receptivity, although the mechanism of ovarian inflammation cannot be ruled out. In presence of pain, the role of surgery has been well-defined but its role especially in asymptomatic women with endometriosis is still to be elucidated. In those women who are having unexplained infertility with mild endometriosis, the treatment of the endometriosis provides a more favorable outcome than the expectant management. Establishing a diagnosis and providing improved chances for conception before IVF will also lead to advances in overall IVF success rates across the board.[4,5]

IMPROVING ACCESS FOR OOCYTE RETRIEVAL

The key indication for managing the "asymptomatic" ovarian endometrioma in patients with subfertility is to improve access for ART. The endometrioma size, location, and transvaginal access for retrieval may all have a factor in determining whether patients require surgery. The accidental spillage during oocyte retrieval is related to high incidence of pelvic infection, so most prefer to go for surgical correction of endometrioma, if it is interfering with ovum pick up. In fact, Hamdan et al. in their meta-analysis found that the outcome of IVF/intracytoplasmic sperm injection (ICSI) did not differ in women who had their endometriomas treated surgically versus no surgery.

TREATING HYDROSALPINX TO IMPROVE IN VITRO FERTILIZATION OUTCOME

Hydrosalpinx might be unilateral or bilateral in those women with endometriosis. The development of hydrosalpinx is mainly due to the anatomical disruption associated with endometriosis. Endometriosis produced an inflammatory state which adds to the development of infertility apart from hydrosalpinx. Many studies have concluded that occlusion of one or both tubes with hydrosalpinx considerably improve the IVF outcome, although the possibility of natural conception has been eliminated.

OVARIAN ENDOMETRIOMA AND SUSPICION OF CONCOMITANT MALIGNANCY

Whenever there is a differential diagnosis of malignancy for a complex adnexal mass, it would be better to go from surgical management. If women are at high risk for ovarian malignancy based on family or personal history, even ovarian endometrioma may present with a difficult diagnosis in them. In such a case, a thorough evaluation of the complex mass is encouraged to determine the overall risk for development of malignancy. Even though most women with endometriotic cyst and endometriosis are considered as a benign condition, there is ever growing interest of study of the relation between endometriosis and epithelial ovarian cancer, thus leading to the need for histologic diagnosis.

CONCOMITANT MANAGEMENT OF DISEASE

In those patients undergoing surgery for conditions other than endometriosis, there may be a concomitant or opportunistic treatment option. In women having uterine fibroid or adenomyosis, the symptoms produced by the same may be mimicking those with endometriosis, for example dysmenorrhea. So, in these women, simultaneous management should be discussed with the patient. But the most important dilemma is the incidental finding of endometriosis in an asymptomatic women. The advantage and disadvantage of surgical interference has to be discussed with the patient and should be carefully considered after weighing the benefits over the risks.

SOCIOCULTURAL AND RELIGIOUS CONSIDERATIONS

The ART options of a patient are strongly influenced by the sociocultural practice and the religious preference. Some religions like Jews, the Roman Catholics, and Islamic Law have different views on the acceptability of different forms of IVF. An open thorough frank discussion between the clinician and the patient has to be carried out to determine whether ART is an acceptable option for the couples. In some cases, surgery may be the only option.

PATIENT CHOICE VERSUS SURGEON CHOICE

The autonomy of the patient takes precedence especially in a patient-centered environment and this part should not be omitted. In an ideal situation, where the couples have access to all sort of treatment options, they should be given the options and they can decide between the medical and surgical alternatives.

Various Surgical Options Available

The various surgical options available prior to ART with respect to ovarian endometrioma include: endometrioma aspiration, endometrioma ablation, and ovarian cystectomy.

Endometrioma Aspiration

Pabuccu et al. studied the effect of endometrioma aspiration prior to controlled ovarian hyperstimulation (COH) in ICSI cycles. As per their observation, the duration of COH was longer in the nonaspirated group. The clinical pregnancy rates and implantation rates were similar in the aspiration versus nonaspiration group. Neither the number of follicles, dosage of gonadotropins, or the number of mature oocytes retrieved vary between the two groups. So, to conclude from their study, since both groups had comparable pregnancy and implantation rates, the aspiration of endometrioma is not of value prior to IVF cycles.[6]

Suzuki et al. studied the outcome of IVF in patients diagnosed with endometriosis with ovarian endometrioma. In their study, they compared three groups of patients, 50 women in each group. In the first group of patients, they have undergone aspiration followed by the examination of aspirated fluid to notify the presence of endometriosis. The second group of patients included who clinically did not have endometriosis but had endometriosis diagnosed laparoscopically. The last group of patients includes those with tubal factor infertility.[7]

From their study, they inferred that ovarian endometrioma did not affect the quality of embryos or lower pregnancy rates. Additionally, the number of mature oocytes retrieved in the first group of patients who had one affected and one normal ovary were comparable, thus demonstrating that endometriosis did not impact oocyte development.[8]

Alternative option is the aspiration of ovarian endometrioma during oocyte retrieval. However, this procedure may place the patient at a higher risk for ovarian or pelvic infection. The theoretical complications associated with this procedure are that, if the chocolate cyst fluid comes into contact with the oocytes, it may contaminate them. However, that has not been supported by a definitive randomized controlled trial (RCT), as large-scale RCTs that examine women affected by ovarian endometriosis do not exist.

Endometrioma Ablation

Another surgical option available is the endometrioma ablation. In the ablation procedure, the cyst wall is destroyed with carbon dioxide (CO_2) laser or bipolar coagulation followed by drainage. This is very frequently done procedure. This procedure is favored by most of infertility specialist with respect to IVF outcomes and is advised as it causes less anatomic distortion and disruption than cystectomy.[9]

Donnez et al. studied the effect of laparoscopic ablation of ovarian endometriotic cysts response to stimulation. Using the CO_2 laser, they vaporized the internal cyst wall. They included those patients in their study who failed to conceive in 1 year following the ablation, at which point IVF was performed. A total of 85 patients were included. Another study group of 289 patients with tubal factor infertility for IVF was included. On comparing the clinical pregnancy, the rates were similar between the two groups. The two groups were statistically comparable across a number of important parameters, including number of dosage and duration of gonadotropin, the number of follicles aspirated, the number of follicles measuring >15 mm in diameter, the number of mature ooctyes aspirated, estradiol (E2) peak levels, fertilization rate, number of embryos/cycle, number of transferred embryos/cycle, implantation rates, and ongoing pregnancy rates.[10,11]

Ovarian Cystectomy

Cystectomy is another surgical alternative available for endometriosis management. The role and effectiveness of cystectomy prior to IVF is a controversial. Among the three surgical options for endometriosis, the lowest recurrence rate is for cystectomy. But the cystectomy has a negative impact on ovarian reserve and ovarian responsiveness to hormonal stimulation. It has been postulated that reduced ovarian response after cystectomy is compensated through increased ovarian stimulation, which results in overall cumulative pregnancy rates that are similar to those of other techniques.

As per Garcia et al, laparoscopic cystectomy performed prior to an IVF cycle did not improve the number of oocytes retrieved, the number of mature oocytes, fertilization rate, and clinical pregnancy rate. Even though laparoscopic cystectomy did not damage ovarian reserve or function, it did not improve the pregnancy rates of patients in a significant manner because ovarian endometriotic cystectomy prior to IVF does not improve pregnancy rates.[12]

Previously, Canis et al. performed a retrospective study to assess ovarian response during IVF cycles after laparoscopic cystectomy. All the endometriotic cyst included in the study measured more than 3 cm. The pregnancy rates during the first cycle of IVF for Group A (endometrioma >3 cm), Group B (no endometrioma), and Group C (tubal infertility) were 35.9%, 31.2%, and 30.5%, respectively. On comparing the three groups, the clinical parameters namely number of oocyte retrieved and the number of embryos attained were almost similar, thus stating that laparoscopic ovarian cystectomy is a beneficial mode of treatment for endometrioma.[13]

Kahyaoglu et al. compared two groups of patients: 22 women who underwent laparoscopic cystectomy and cauterization before IVF and 22 women with tubal factor infertility who proceeded directly to IVF. In the cystectomy group, fewer follicles and oocytes were retrieved than the endometrioma operated group. The clinical pregnancy rate in the endometrioma group exceeded that of the tubal factor group by 9%, with rates of 45% and 36%, respectively. When comparing the operated and contralateral normal ovary, the normal ovary was producing more mature follicles for retrieval than the affected one.[14]

When combining cystectomy by stripping with ablation through a CO_2 laser, it may have favorable results in preserving ovarian reserve. Although this is a laparoscopic modification of traditional cystectomy, it is effective and has immense potential for future development.[15] The ablated portion is proximal to the ovarian hilum and thus, vaporization is the preferred technique for this location as it contains the vasculature most prone to damage in the ovary.

To improve the success rate in women with endometrioma, she should first undergo treatment to minimize the presence of disease. Although laparoscopic surgery has long been considered the first-line treatment for minimal and mild (stage I and II) endometriosis, a newer approach claims that surgery may not be beneficial in terms of pregnancy rates and disease management if the ovarian endometriomas <3 cm in diameter. Nevertheless, it is noteworthy that for patients who do not require IVF and want to try naturally, surgery may be their best option as Donnez et al. 2004 reported a postoperative pregnancy rate as high as 50%. While the surgical technique that yields the best results for IVF is still being debated, a careful review of recent studies shows that laparoscopic removal of ovarian endometriomas that are less than <3 cm in diameter has no much effect on pregnancy rates naturally or with IVF and may in fact it can cause irreparable damage to the affected ovary. So, surgery to be considered in only those with cysts which are large and painful or when medical therapy fails or to exclude the diagnosis of malignancy.

HYDROSALPINGES AND IN VITRO FERTILIZATION

Due to the anatomic alterations being associated with endometriosis, one may develop concurrent unilateral or bilateral hydrosalpinges, and the inflammatory mediators related to endometriosis diminish the IVF success rate. At present, several studies support the view that removal or occlusion of the tubes may eliminate the possibility of natural conception but may improve the IVF outcomes by nearly 50%.

SURGERY AND EXPERTISE

Surgery must be performed carefully to keep to a minimum any damage to the ovary (by excision or ablative technique). To achieve this, experienced surgeons and an appropriate technique are required. The level of expertise in endometriosis surgery inversely correlates with the amount of ovarian tissue inadvertently removed together with the endometrioma wall. Indeed, the experience of the surgeon may affect the live birth rate after IVF in women with surgically removed endometriomas.

DEMERITS OF SURGICAL MODALITY

- Ovarian reserve may be lower in women with ovarian endometrioma compared with those women without.
- Surgical excision of an endometrioma is ideal for pain but may lead to reduced ovarian reserve in the short term.
- Bilateral, compared to unilateral, ovarian cystectomy for endometriomas may result in a greater negative effect on ovarian reserve.
- Recurrent endometrioma excision may further reduce ovarian reserve compared with primary surgery.

The couple has to be well-counseled in detail regarding the pros and cons about the surgical treatment available and the various necessity of surgery before ART. Based on a proper consensus from the couple, we can decide on the future treatment modality.

CONCLUSION

- Infertility is commonly associated with endometriosis.
- The role of surgery for endometriosis-related subfertility may be considered in those with hydrosalpinges undergoing IVF, management of ovarian endometriomas in specific circumstances, and when a patient requests surgery as an alternative to ART.
- Before ART, the role for surgery includes: improving the access for oocyte retrieval and management of hydrosalpinx.
- The various surgical options available prior to ART with respect to ovarian endometrioma include: endometrioma aspiration, endometrioma ablation, and ovarian cystectomy.
- Surgery for ovarian endometriomas requires special attention due to the risk of potential harm on future fertility.
- Surgical expertise greatly influences the management, especially when considering the ovarian reserve.

REFERENCES

1. Barnhart K, Dunsmoor-Su R, Coutifaris C. Effect of endometriosis on in vitro fertilization. Fertil Steril. 2002; 77(6):1148-55.
2. Marcoux S, Maheux R, Bérubé S. Laparoscopic surgery in infertile women with minimal or mild endometriosis. Canadian Collaborative Group on Endometriosis. N Engl J Med. 1997;337(4):217-22.
3. Kodama H, Fukuda J, Karube H, et al. Benefit of in vitro fertilization treatment for endometriosis-associated infertility. Fertil Steril. 1996;66(6):974-9.
4. Opøien HK, Fedorcsak P, Omland AK, et al. In vitro fertilization is a successful treatment in endometriosis-associated infertility. Fertil Steril. 2012;97(4):912-8.
5. Tsoumpou I, Kyrgiou M, Gelbaya TA, et al. The effect of surgical treatment for endometrioma on in vitro fertilization outcomes: a systematic review and meta-analysis. Fertil Steril. 2009;92(1):75-87.
6. Pabuccu R, Onalan G, Goktolga U, et al. Aspiration of ovarian endometriomas before intracytoplasmic sperm injection. Fertil Steril. 2004;82(3):705-11.
7. Suzuki T, Izumi S, Matsubayashi H, et al. Impact of ovarian endometrioma on oocytes and pregnancy outcome in in vitro fertilization. Fertil Steril. 2005;83(4):908-13.
8. Yaron Y, Peyser MR, Samuel D, et al. Infected endometriotic cysts secondary to oocyte aspiration for in-vitro fertilization. Hum Reprod. 1994;9(9):1759-60.
9. Shimizu Y, Takashima A, Takahashi K, et al. Long-term outcome, including pregnancy rate, recurrence rate and ovarian reserve, after laparoscopic laser ablation surgery in infertile women with endometrioma. J Obstet Gynaecol Res. 2010;36(1):115-8.
10. Donnez J, Wyns C, Nisolle M. Does ovarian surgery for endometriomas impair the ovarian response to gonadotropin? Fertil Steril. 2001;76(4):662-5.
11. Donnez J, Pirard C, Smets M, et al. Surgical management of endometriosis. Best Pract Res Clin Obstet Gynaecol. 2004;18(2):329-48.
12. Garcia-Velasco JA, Mahutte NG, Corona J, et al. Removal of endometriomas before in vitro fertilization does not improve fertility outcomes: a matched, case-control study. Fertil Steril. 2004;81(5):1194-7.
13. Canis M, Pouly JL, Tamburro S, et al. Ovarian response during IVF-embryo transfer cycles after laparoscopic ovarian cystectomy for endometriotic cysts of >3 cm in diameter. Hum Reprod. 2001;16(12):2583-6.
14. Kahyaoglu S, Ertas E, Kahyaoglu I, et al. Does laparoscopic cystectomy and cauterization of endometriomas greater than 3 cm diminish ovarian response to controlled ovarian hyperstimulation during IVF-ET? A case-control study. J Obstet Gynaecol Res. 2008;34(6):1010-3.
15. Donnez J, Lousse JC, Jadoul P, et al. Laparoscopic management of endometriomas using a combined technique of excisional (cystectomy) and ablative surgery. Fertil Steril. 2010;94(1):28-32.

Index

Page numbers followed by *b* refer to box, *f* refer to figure, *fc* refer to flowchart, and *t* refer to table.

A

Abscess 63
Adenomyoma
    large 27*f*
    removal of 27
Adenomyomectomy, laparoscopic 27*f*
Adenomyosis 17, 24, 26, 27, 37, 74
    effect of 25
    focal 25*f*, 27
    large focal 25*f*
Adhesiolysis 44
Adhesion prevention 45
Alcohol consumption 63
American College of Obstetricians and Gynecologists 9*fc*
American Reproductive Society 13
American Society for Reproductive Medicine 13, 30
    classification of Müllerian anomalies 30
Anastrozole 68
Androgens 63
Angiogenesis inhibitors 68
Antiangiogenesis factors 21
Anti-inflammatory agents 68
Anti-Müllerian hormone 58
    serum 38
Antioxidants 68
Antiretroviral therapy 17
Antral follicle count 38
Anxiety 6
Aromatase 3
    inhibitors 20, 68
Assisted reproductive technology 15, 24, 37, 53, 70, 73
Autoimmune theory 49

B

Biochemical tests 13
Biomolecular theory 2
Bladder 46, 50, 51
    endometriosis of 46*f*, 49, 52, 53
Blood, collection of 25*f*
Bone mineral density 9
Bowel
    disease 7
    endometriosis 42, 46
    preparations 51
    wall infiltration, depth of 51

C

Cabergoline quinagolide 68
Cancer antigen 7
Carbon dioxide 75
Carcinoma 63
Cells
    contractile nonmuscle 49
    endometrial 49
Cervical
    agenesis 30
    anomaly 29
    aplasia 29
        unilateral 29
    dysgenesis 30
Cervix
    distension of 31
    double normal 29
    normal 29
Cesarean section 62, 63
Cetrorelix acetate 68
Coelomic metaplasia 1
    Meyer and Ivanoff theory of 2
    theory 48, 62
Coital function 66
Conservative uterine, role of 27
Constipation 7
Contraceptives pill
    combined
        hormonal 18
        oral 8, 18, 63, 69
    oral 6, 19, 26, 39
Controlled ovarian hyperstimulation 75
Corpus
    luteal cyst 14
    luteum 67
Cyclooxygenase 68
Cyst 63
    complex 14, 14*f*
    enucleation 44*f*
    hemorrhagic 14, 67
    management, endometrial 10
    myometrial 25*f*
    ovarian 15
Cystadenoma 67
Cystectomy 75
    endometriotic 44, 45*fc*
    ovarian 38, 75
Cystitis, recurrent 51
Cytochrome P450 3

D

D-amino acid 69
Danazol 20, 26, 68
Deep infiltrating endometriosis 42*f*, 43, 43*f*, 48, 50, 53, 54, 69
    classification of 53, 54
    intestinal 49, 53
    retroperitoneal 50*f*

Depomedroxyprogesterone acetate 9, 68
Depression 6
Dermoid 67
    cyst 67
Diarrhea 7, 49
Dienogest 9, 67, 68*t*
Diethylstilbestrol 30
Direct implantation theory 2
Dopamine receptor 2 agonists 21
Doppler ultrasound 67
Dr David experience 35*fc*
Drosophila, Ortholog of 4
Dyschezia 49-51
Dysfunction, endometrial 66
Dysmenorrhea 26, 42, 49-51
    severe 43, 51
Dyspareunia 6, 42, 49-51, 66
    deep 43, 51

E

Elagolix 68
Embryo freezing 59, 60
Embryonic cell rest 1
Endogenous anti-angiogenic activity 21
Endometrioma 9, 11, 14*f*, 15*f*, 32, 33, 44, 48, 58, 60, 67, 70, 76
    ablation 75
    aspiration 75
    atypical features of 67, 67*t*
    bilateral 44, 58, 70
    externa 62
    left-sided 1*f*, 10
    multiple 14*f*
    right ovarian 33*f*
    typical USG features of 67, 67*t*
Endometriosis 1, 2*f*, 6, 7, 8*f*, 13, 17, 18, 21, 29-32, 35, 37-40, 42, 46, 48, 49, 52, 58-60, 62, 66, 67, 70, 73, 74, 77
    abdominal wall 62
    adolescent 6, 9*fc*
    associated infertility 14, 15
    bilateral ovarian 49
    challenges in 37
    clinical features of 66*b*
    course of 7
    cutaneous 62
    deep 40, 48, 51
        invasive 48
    development of 48
    diagnosis of 1, 11, 66
    endopelvic 62
    etiopathogenesis of 1
    excise deep 44

extraovarian 67
histological diagnosis of 63
ideal protocol for 38
impact of 58
in vitro fertilization outcomes in 59
infiltrative 14
isolated deep 48
lesions 49
main sites for 42
majority of 14
mechanical cause of 31
medical management of 17
medications used in 18b
mild 2f, 44
mild-to-moderate 73
minimal 44
moderate 44
natural course of 7
pathogenesis of 1, 2
pathophysiology of 18b
prevalence of 6, 48
rectosigmoid 48
rectovaginal 42, 67
recurrence 40
retrocervical 42, 46
retroperitoneal 48
severe 44
stage of 38
suppression of 38
symptoms of 6, 63
theories of 2
treatment of 12, 19
types of 48
ureteric 49, 53
Endometriotic
  cells, lymphovascular dissemination of 3f
  cyst 73
    differential diagnosis of 67, 67t
    drainage of 10f
  implants 17
    ablation of 43
  lesions 21, 50
Endometrium, germinal epithelia of 48
Enigmatic disease 42
Environment theory 3
Episiotomy 62
Equine estrogens, conjugated 11
Estradiol 69
Estrogen 18
  dependent disease, benign 48
  formation, inhibition of 68
Estrogenic receptor isoforms 4
Etanercept 68
Etonogestrel implant 20
European Society of Gastrointestinal Endoscopy 29
European Society of Human Reproduction and Embryology 29, 70

F

Fallopian tubes 62
Fertility
  preservation 59
    cost-benefit analysis of 60
    options of 59
    technology 58
  preserving surgery 27, 59
  prevention 58
  sparing
    surgery 27
    treatment 24
Fertilization 3
Fine-needle aspiration cytology 63
Follicle-stimulating hormone 19, 58, 69
Food and Drug Administration 68t, 69

G

Galactose-1-phosphate uridyltransferase 30
Gastrointestinal symptoms 6, 51
Genes
  angiogenic 21
  anti-inflammatory 21
Genetic theory 2
Genital tract anomalies, female 29
Gestrinone 68
Glands 48
  endometrial 1, 49, 63
Gonadotropin-releasing hormone 9, 18, 26, 67, 68
  agonist 8, 19, 38, 39, 67, 69t, 73
    therapy 26
  analogs 63
  antagonists 19, 68
Goserelin 68
  acetate 69
Granule 63
Granulosa cells, ovarian 68
Ground glass homogeneous echoes 14f

H

Halban's theory 2
Heavy menstrual flow 63
Hematocolpometra 31
Hematocolpos 31
Hematoma 63
Hematometra 33, 33f
  laparoscopic view of 33f
  ultrasonography of 33f
Hemiuterus 29
Hemorrhage 14, 15
Hemosiderin-Laden macrophages 1
Herlyn-Werner-Wunderlich syndrome 32, 32f
  magnetic resonance imaging of 33f
Hilus sign 67
Hormone
  luteinizing 19, 69
  therapy 69
    combination 9

Hydronephrosis 51, 52
Hydrosalpinx 74
  development of 74
Hyperechogenic wall 67
Hypoplasia 29
Hypothalamic-pituitary-ovarian axis 67
Hysterectomy 62
  early 63
Hysterolaparoscopy, combined 32

I

Iliac spine, anterior superior 42
Imperforate hymen 29
Implantation
  failure 4
  impaired 38
In vitro fertilization 37, 67, 73, 76
  cycle 59
  outcome 59, 74
Incision hernia 63
Infertility 25, 37, 50, 66, 77
Infliximab 68
International Ovarian Tumor Analysis 14
Intestine 50
Intracytoplasmic sperm injection 39, 67, 74
Intrauterine insemination 15, 40, 67
Ipsilateral renal agenesis 32
  syndrome 30
Isoflavones 68

K

Kissing ovaries, bilateral 42f

L

Labor, spontaneous onset of 63
L-amino acid, substitution of 69
Laparoscopy 1f, 31, 37, 42, 73
  advantages of 9
  diagnostic 7
Laparotomy 62
Lesions, hourglass-shaped 50
Letrozole 39, 68
Leuprolide 68
  acetate 69
Levonorgestrel intrauterine
  device 68
  system 8, 19
Lipoma 63
Low ovarian reserve 38
Lower urinary tract symptoms 51
Lymphatic spread, Halban's theory of 2
Lymphoma 63

M

Macrophages 66
Magnetic resonance imaging 31, 37, 50, 52, 67
Malignancy, risk of 64
Mass

Index

abdominal 31
    oval 67
Mayer-Rokitansky-Küster-Hauser syndrome 32, 34
Medroxyprogesterone 19
Melatonin 68
Menses, irregular 6
Menstrual bleeding 51
Mesothelial cells 2
Metalloproteinase 3
Meyer and Ivanoff theory 2
Mifepristone 68
Migraine 6
Müllerian agenesis 32
Müllerian anomalies 6, 7, 29-31, 33, 35
    classification of 29t
    higher incidence of 30
    incidence of 34
    nonobstructive 31
    obstructive 30
    prevalence of 30
    range of 29
Müllerian defects 30
Müllerian duct 29
    anomalies 29
Müllerian malformations 31
Müllerian remnant 2
    theory 3
Müllerian structures, abnormal 31
Musculoskeletal disorders 7
Myofibroblasts 49
Myometrium, adjacent 24

N

Nafarelin 68
    acetate 69
Nausea 7
Nerves
    retroperitoneal 53
    sparing surgery, nerve dissection for 45f
Neuroma 63
Nodules
    endometriotic 44
    excised rectovaginal 43f
Nonsteroidal anti-inflammatory drugs 7-9, 18, 67, 68
Norethindrone acetate 9, 11, 68, 69

O

Obstructed hemivagina, ipsilateral renal agenesis syndrome 30, 32
Oocyte
    freezing 59, 60, 67
    retrieval 59, 74
        risk of 60
Oral lichen planus 68
Ovarian
    cortex 70
        freezing 60

endometrioma 10, 10f, 70, 74, 77
    asymptomatic 74
    differential diagnosis of 67, 67t
    management of 73
hyperstimulation syndrome 39
inflammation, mechanism of 74
reserve 38, 58
stimulation 40, 59
Ovary 62
    endometrioma of 10, 42, 44, 44f
    germinal epithelia of 48
Ovulation suppressing agents 68
Ovulatory dysfunction 66
Ovum pick up 66

P

Pain 45
    abdominal 7
    killers 6
    rectal 49
    severe
        chronic 51
        hypogastric 51
Papillae, absence of 67
Papillary projections 67
Parenchyma, ovarian 67
Peculiar atypical red vascular lesions 8f
Pelvic
    adhesions 44
    endometriosis 62
    mass 6
    organs 13
    pain 18, 32, 37, 42
        chronic 6, 42, 43, 50
Pelvis
    final appearance of 44f
    MRI of 51
Pentoxifylline 21, 68
Peptidoglycan 68
Peripheral estrogen levels 40
Peritoneal endometriosis 42, 48
    fulguration of 44f
Peritoneal windows 8f
Peritoneum 62
    germinal epithelia of 48
Peritubal adhesions 66
Periureteral vessels 53
Phagocytosis 66
Phytoestrogens 68
Polycystic ovaries 30
Poor oocyte quality 38
Posterior wall fornix lesions 50, 50f
Pouch of Douglas 2, 13, 44, 49-52, 62
Pregnancy loss, recurrent 30
Progesterone 18, 69
    containing contraceptives 19
    receptor antagonists 68
Progestins 9, 68
Progestogens 63

Progressive estrogen-dependent disease 48
Prostaglandins 7
Protein kinase, mitogen-activated 4

R

Radical surgery 53
Raloxifene 68
Ramakrishna experience 35fc
Randomized controlled trial 39, 75
Rectal
    aqueous contrast 51
    evaluation 52
    excision 45
    mobilization 43f
    mucosa 52
    submucosa 52
Rectovaginal nodule, excision of 43f
Rectovaginal septum
    endometriosis of 44, 45f
    lesions 50
Rectovaginal space 51
Rectum 45
Renal agenesis 30
Retrograde menstruation 48
    Sampson's theory of 2
Retroperitoneal lesions, subclassification of 50
Robert's uterus 33
    hysteroscopic
        resection of 34f
        view of 34f
    laparoscopic view of 34f
    magnetic resonance imaging of 34f
    relook hysteroscopic view of 34f
    ultrasonography of 33f

S

Saline, normal 42
Sampson's theory 2, 48, 62
Scar endometriosis 62, 64
    therapy of 63
Selective estrogen receptor modulator 11, 68
Selective progesterone receptor modulators 20, 68
Septa 67
    fibrin 14
Septate
    cervix 29
    uterus 29, 30, 34
Septostomy 32
Simvastatin 68
Soft tissue sarcoma 63
Sonography
    high-frequency 52
    transvaginal 1f, 14, 67
Sperm inactivation 66
Statins 21
Stroma 1, 48
    leads 49
Subfertility 6

Surface endometriosis 48
    electrocoagulation 9f
Surgery 70
    conservative 26, 53
    endometriotic 42
    laparoscopic 62
Surgical therapy
    advantages of 70t
    disadvantages of 70t

T

Tanner system 7
Tenesmus 49
Thromboembolism, risk of 18
Tissue
    adenomyomatous 27
    adenomyotic 27
    endometrial 48, 67
    endometriotic 32
    ovarian 58
Torus uterinus 49
Transverse vaginal septum 29, 30
Triptorelin 69
Tubal motility 66
Tubes, anatomical distortion of 66
Tumor necrosis factor 3
    alpha blockers 21

U

Ultra-long protocol 38
Ultrasonography 63, 67
    three-dimensional 31, 67
    transrectal 50-52
Ureter, endometriosis of 42, 46, 53
Ureteral involvement 49, 52
Ureteric dissection 43f
Urinary bladder, endometriosis of 42, 46
Urinary tract
    disease 51
    endometriosis 48
Uterine
    agenesis 30
    anomaly 29
        nonobstructive 31
    cavity 27, 48
    didelphys 33f
    fibroid 74
    incision 27
Uterosacral ligament 1, 2f, 45, 49-53, 62
Uterovaginal agenesis 29
Uterus
    arcuate 29, 30
    asymmetric
        dissection of 27
        enlarged 25
    bicornuate 29, 34
    bicorporeal 29
    carina of 49
    didelphys 29, 30, 32, 34
    distension of 31
    dysmorphic 29
    normal 29
    right horn of 33f
    unicornuate 29, 30, 34

V

Vagina 50, 51
    distension of 31
    normal 29
Vaginal
    agenesis 30
    anomaly 29
    aplasia 29
    excision 43
    fornix, posterior 49
    injection 51
    septa 31
    septum, longitudinal
        nonobstructing 29
        obstructing 29
Valproic acid 68
Vascular
    dissemination theory 48
    endothelial growth factor 3
    theory 2

www.ingramcontent.com/pod-product-compliance
Ingram Content Group UK Ltd.
Pitfield, Milton Keynes, MK11 3LW, UK
UKHW052230140425
457402UK00006B/39